Emergency Care of the
Patient with a Heart Attack

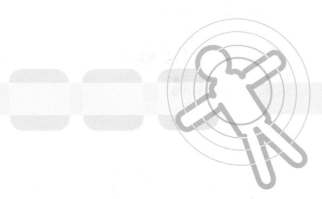

To our partners Karen, Chris and Jane, for
supporting us through this and everything
we do.

For Elsevier:
Commissioning Editor: Susan Young
Development Editor: Catherine Jackson
Production Manager: Joannah Duncan
Design: Stewart Larking
Illustrator: Chartwell Illustrators

Emergency Care of the Patient with a Heart Attack

Roger Gamon RN BA(Hons)
Primary PCI Clinical Project Manager,
Greater Manchester & Cheshire Cardiac Network, UK

Tom Quinn MPhil RN FESC FRCN
Professor of Cardiac Nursing, Faculty of Health and Life Sciences,
Coventry University, Coventry, UK; Clinical Lead, Cardiovascular
Diseases, National Library for Health

Brian Parr BA(Hons) Dip(N) RN
Nurse Clinician (Acute Coronary Syndromes and Angina),
Cardiology Department, Salford Royal Hospital Trust, Salford, UK

Foreword
Malcolm Woollard MPH MA(Ed) MBA Dip IMC (RCSEd) PGCE RN
SRPara FASI ILTM
Consultant Paramedic and Director, Faculty of Pre-hospital Care
Research Unit, Department of Academic Emergency Medicine
The James Cook University Hospital, Middlesbrough;
Visiting Professor in Pre-hospital Emergency Care, University of
Teeside

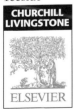

CHURCHILL LIVINGSTONE

ELSEVIER

EDINBURGH LONDON NEW YORK OXFORD PHILADELPHIA ST LOUIS SYDNEY TORONTO 2007

CHURCHILL
LIVINGSTONE
ELSEVIER

© 2007, Elsevier Limited. All rights reserved.
First published 2007

ISBN-13: 9780443102493
ISBN-10: 0 443 10249 X

British Library Cataloguing in Publication Data
A catalogue record for this book is available from the British Library.

Library of Congress Cataloging in Publication Data
A catalog record for this book is available from the Library of Congress.

Note
Knowledge and best practice in this field are constantly changing. As new research and experience broaden our knowledge, changes in practice, treatment and drug therapy may become necessary or appropriate. Readers are advised to check the most current information provided (i) on procedures featured or (ii) by the manufacturer of each product to be administered, to verify the recommended dose or formula, the method and duration of administration, and contraindications. It is the responsibility of the practitioner, relying on their own experience and knowledge of the patient, to make diagnoses, to determine dosages and the best treatment for each individual patient, and to take all appropriate safety precautions. To the fullest extent of the law, neither the Publisher nor the Authors assume any liability for any injury and/or damage to persons or property arising out of or related to any use of the material contained in this book.

The Publisher

ELSEVIER
your source for books,
journals and multimedia
in the health sciences

www.elsevierhealth.com

Working together to grow
libraries in developing countries
www.elsevier.com | www.bookaid.org | www.sabre.org

ELSEVIER   BOOK AID International   Sabre Foundation

The
publisher's
policy is to use
paper manufactured
from sustainable forests

Printed in China

Contents

Foreword by Professor Malcolm Woollard   vii

Abbreviations   ix

Trial Acronyms   xi

Chapter 1. Emergency care of the heart attack patient – an overview 3

Chapter 2. Assessing the patient with chest pain or discomfort 17

Chapter 3. Immediate management 27

Chapter 4. Recording a 12-lead ECG 35

Chapter 5. Interpreting the 12-lead ECG in the patient with suspected ACS 45

Chapter 6. Complications 65

Chapter 7. Cardiac rhythm disturbances and ACS . . . 75

Chapter 8. Reperfusion 1: Thrombolytic treatment for STEMI 101

Chapter 9. Care during administration of thrombolytic treatment 115

Chapter 10. Reperfusion 2: Interventional cardiology in the treatment of the patient with STEMI 123

Chapter 11. The non-STEMI patient with ACS 133

Chapter 12. Measuring and improving the quality of emergency cardiac care 153

Index   161

Foreword

Acute coronary syndromes remain a leading cause of death in the Western World. In the UK alone, a quarter of a million individuals will suffer a myocardial infarction each year: up to a third of these will die before reaching hospital. Of those that live enough to be admitted, a further 8 to 13% will die. But this is just the tip of the iceberg: UK Emergency Departments will see over 700 000 patient episodes each year relating to chest pain or associated problems. All of these patients are someone's mother, father, wife, husband, partner, son, daughter, or friend. All will have contributed to society, and all have the potential to continue to do so.

The only hope of reducing the significant impact on society of acute coronary syndromes is appropriate (that is, evidence-based) clinical intervention without delay, including early defibrillation and early reperfusion therapy. The distinguished authors of this book have addressed this aspiration by drawing on their extensive clinical, academic, and management expertise to describe and summarise the initial diagnosis and care of this deserving group of patients. This highly accessible and lucid text will meet the learning needs of a variety of health care practitioners working in a range of settings. Its brevity encourages it to be read from cover to cover (I managed this in only two hours) but the content is also sufficiently detailed to provide a wealth of current references to encourage up-to-date evidence-based practice.

This book covers the diagnosis and management of acute coronary syndromes, from system design, through initial interventions, recording and interpretation of 12-lead ECGs, choosing a reperfusion strategy, treatment of complications (including heart failure, cardiac arrest, and arrhythmias), and clinical governance. Stressing the key considerations to be made at every point, it emphasises that the priorities for care are the same regardless of whether the patient is being managed in or out of hospital.

This is an essential introductory text for those new to the emergency care of patients with acute coronary syndromes, but it will also provide an excellent update on the latest evidence-based practice for those returning to this clinical specialty or for experienced practitioners in need of a refresher.

Professor Malcolm Woollard MPH MBA MA(Ed)
Dip IMC (RCSEd) PGCE RN SRPara FASI
Consultant Paramedic and Director, Faculty of
Pre-hospital Care Research Unit, Middlesbrough;
Visiting Professor in Pre-hospital Emergency Care,
University Of Teesside.
UK, 2007

Abbreviations

ACS	acute coronary syndrome
AMI	acute myocardial infarction
APTT	activated partial thromboplastin time
AV	atrioventricular
BBB	bundle branch block
BP	blood pressure
CABG	coronary artery bypass graft
CAD	coronary artery disease
CCU	cardiac care unit
CHD	coronary heart disease
COPD	chronic obstructive pulmonary disease
ECG	electrocardiogram
GTN	glyceryl trinitrate
ICH	intracranial haemorrhage
IV	intravenous
LBBB	left bundle branch block
LMWH	low-molecular-weight heparin
MI	myocardial infarction
NSF	National Service Framework
NSTEMI	non-ST segment elevation myocardial infarction
PCI	percutaneous coronary intervention
PEA	pulseless electrical activity
RBBB	right bundle branch block
RCA	right coronary artery
RVI	right ventricular infarction
STEMI	ST segment elevation myocardial infarction
VF	ventricular fibrillation
VT	ventricular tachycardia

Trial Acronyms

ASSENT	Assessment of the Safety and Efficacy of a New Thrombolytic
CRUSADE	Can Rapid risk stratification of Unstable angina patients Suppress ADverse outcomes with Early implementation of the ACC/AHA Guidelines?
EMMACE	Evaluation of Methods and Management of Acute Coronary Events
GRACE	Global Registry of Acute Coronary Events
GUSTO	Global Utilization of Streptokinase and T-pa for Occluded coronary arteries
ISIS	International Study of Infarct Survival

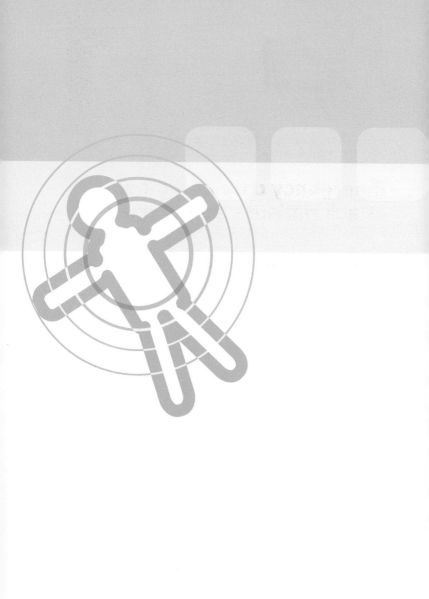

Chapter 1

Emergency care of the heart attack patient – an overview

Chapter contents

Introduction	4
Timely defibrillation saves lives	6
Timely reperfusion saves lives	7
Saving time saves lives	7
Pre-hospital treatment saves time – and lives	9
Systems delay – updating the '4Ds' concept	9
Pharmacological or mechanical treatment of MI?	11
Non-STEMI presentations	11
Summary	11

This chapter:

- Defines the term 'heart attack', or acute coronary syndrome (ACS)

- Sets ACS care in the context of the burden of cardiovascular diseases in the UK

- Outlines the key pathophysiology

- Sets out the key treatments for patients with suspected or confirmed ACS

- Highlights the importance of reducing delay from symptom onset to treatment.

Introduction

The term 'heart attack' can mean many different things to patients and families and to health professionals and is generally taken to represent a myocardial infarction (MI). The definition of MI is derived from a consensus statement of the main professional societies across Europe and the United States and relates to the presence of a combination of changes in the 12-lead electrocardiogram (ECG) and markers of myocardial necrosis (Fig. 1.1). This definition is subject to continuing evaluation (Fox et al 2004).

Acute coronary syndrome (ACS) is an umbrella term that describes a spectrum of conditions – including MI – sharing a common underlying pathophysiology: obstruction of coronary blood flow due to thrombus following disruption of coronary artery plaque (Fig. 1.2). The main classifications of ACS relate to changes in the ECG and release of markers of myocardial necrosis: ST segment elevation MI (STEMI), non-ST segment elevation MI (NSTEMI) and unstable angina (Fig. 1.3).

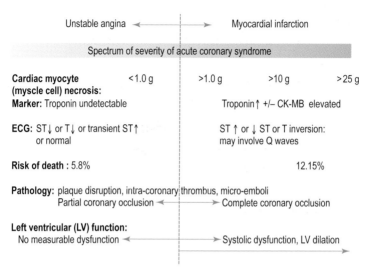

Figure 1. 1 Acute coronary syndrome (ACS) ranges from unstable angina without detectable cardiac muscle damage to extensive myocardial infarction (MI). Reproduced with permission from Fox (2004).

An ACS diagnosis carries a significant mortality risk. In patients who reach hospital alive, mortality at six months is 12% in STEMI patients and 8% in those with unstable angina. It is important to recognise that patients with NSTEMI presentations have the highest mortality of the three categories, with 13% dead at six months (Fox 2004).

The burden of disease

The British Heart Foundation (2004) estimate that each year over a quarter of a million MIs occur in the UK. There are over a million survivors of MI in the UK, and approximately 892 000 people aged 45 years or more living with heart failure, often a consequence of delayed reperfusion. Goodacre et al (2005) estimate that 700 000 emergency department attendances in England and Wales annually are due to chest pain and related complaints. The burden on health services is therefore substantial.

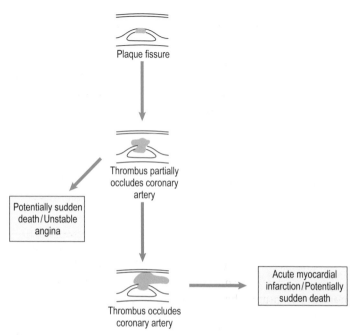

Figure 1.2 Occluded coronary artery.

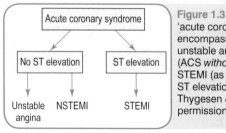

Figure 1.3 The umbrella term 'acute coronary syndrome' (ACS) encompasses the diagnoses of unstable angina and NSTEMI (ACS *without* ST elevation) and STEMI (as the term implies, *with* ST elevation). Adapted from Alpert, Thygesen & Antman (2000), with permission from ACC.

Timely defibrillation saves lives

Many deaths from MI occur before the patient reaches hospital. Standards and guidelines are predicated on evidence that survival from cardiac arrest is more likely in the presence of a trained responder equipped with a defibrillator. In the United Kingdom Heart Attack Study, 40% of cardiac arrest patients survived to 30 days if their arrest occurred in the presence of an ambulance crew, compared to 2–8% of patients whose arrest was witnessed by a bystander (Norris 1998).

Timely reperfusion saves lives

The 'mega trials' of thrombolytic treatment in the 1980s demonstrated that the sooner patients with MI were treated with a thrombolytic agent the better their chances of survival. That aspirin was effective in reducing mortality was also demonstrated. Most benefit in patients treated with thrombolysis is seen within the first ('golden') hour following symptom onset (Boersma et al 1996). The importance of very early treatment has been demonstrated to apply to both pharmacological (thrombolytic) and mechanical (percutaneous coronary intervention (PCI)) reperfusion techniques. Immediate PCI to treat acute MI is becoming increasingly common in the UK and offers advantages over thrombolysis in terms of reduced bleeding risk in particular. The key imperative is, of course, to attempt to restore coronary flow using whichever strategy is promptly available. Thrombolysis remains a viable alternative to PCI, certainly within the first three hours of onset (Silber et al 2005).

Saving time saves lives

The National Service Framework (NSF) for coronary heart disease (CHD) (Department of Health 2000) set national standards for improved prevention and treatment of heart disease in England. For patients with STEMI or (presumed) new left bundle branch block (LBBB) on the 12-lead ECG, the NSF

BOX: **1.1** |||||||||||||||||||||||||||||||||||||||||||||||||||||||||||||||||||||||||||||||||||||||||

NSF standards for acute coronary syndromes
(Department of Health 2000)

Standard five
People with symptoms of a possible heart attack should receive help from an individual equipped with and appropriately trained in the use of a defibrillator within eight minutes of calling for help, to maximise the benefits of resuscitation should it be necessary.

Standard six
People thought to be suffering from a heart attack should be assessed professionally and, if indicated, receive aspirin. Thrombolysis should be given within 60 minutes of calling for professional help.

Standard seven
NHS Trusts should put in place agreed protocols/systems of care so that people admitted to hospital with proven heart attack are assessed appropriately and offered treatments of proven clinical and cost effectiveness to reduce their risk of disability and death.

sets three standards (Box 1.1). Other UK countries have set similar standards (National Assembly for Wales 2001, Scottish Executive 2002).

Both the American Heart Association (AHA) and the European Society of Cardiology (ESC) recommend the use of primary PCI for patients presenting with STEMI where the delay from first medical contact to balloon is 90 minutes or less (Van de Werf et al 2003, Antman et al 2004). Primary PCI is also preferred – if facilities are available – in the following scenarios:

- cardiogenic shock

- heart failure (Killip class ≥ 3 (see Chapter 6, p. 67))

- contraindications to thrombolysis
- late presentation (symptom onset > 3 hours ago)
- where diagnosis of STEMI is in doubt (Antman et al 2004).

Pre-hospital treatment saves time – and lives

A meta-analysis demonstrated a 17% reduction in all-cause mortality in patients given pre-hospital thrombolysis (Morrison et al 2000). Keeling et al (2003) reported that autonomous paramedic pre-hospital thrombolysis was feasible and safe and associated with improved 'call-to-needle' times. Pedley et al (2003) reported that treatment times improved markedly when pre-hospital thrombolysis was available. Thousands of patients in the UK have received thrombolysis from a paramedic since the NSF was published. Direct transfer for primary PCI is also increasingly available to treat MI patients.

Meta-analysis has shown the availability of a 12-lead ECG in an ambulance reduces delays and improves care for patients with MI (Ioannidis et al 2001), although the added value of ECG telemetry transmission may depend on the particular system employed (Woollard et al 2005). Patient safety should be safeguarded by agreeing roles and responsibilities regarding advice given (e.g. by hospital staff) and actions taken (by paramedics) (Quinn et al 2002).

Systems delay: updating the '4 Ds' concept

The National Heart Attack Alert Program (1994) in the United States proposed a model for reducing delay to heart attack treatment: the '4 Ds':

- **D1, Door** – initial triage based on a rapid assessment of the patient and handover from ambulance staff if the patient came by ambulance

- **D2, Data** – time from arrival to recording the first 12-lead ECG

- **D3, Decision** – time from arrival to an appropriate clinician interpreting ECG and other data, explaining the risks and benefits to the patient and ordering thrombolysis, and

- **D4, Drug** – time from decision to administer thrombolysis to actually starting the treatment, including locating and drawing up the drug.

An extension of the model – D0, Domicile – to encompass pre-hospital delays was proposed by Quinn and Thompson (1995).

Recent guidelines have introduced the concept of a 'contact to thrombolysis' time of no more than 30 min from the patient either arriving at hospital or having initial contact with a paramedic. For primary PCI the equivalent proposed standard is contact to balloon inflation within 90 min (Antman et al 2004).

Patient delay

There is little evidence that media or public education interventions reduce delay and there is some evidence that such campaigns result in an increase in emergency calls and hospital attendances in patients without ACS (Kainth et al 2004). Efforts might be better focused on educating higher-risk patient groups such as survivors of a previous ACS event and those with established CHD.

Pharmacological or mechanical treatment of MI?

A meta-analysis of trials comparing PCI to hospital thrombolysis suggested lower death rates in the PCI patients, who also had less adverse events including haemorrhagic stroke and the need for repeat angiography than patients who received thrombolysis (Keeley et al 2003). PCI may reduce overall costs compared to thrombolysis in patients who are within one hour's travel time of a hospital able to provide this intervention (Machecourt et al 2005). The mortality benefit of primary PCI over hospital thrombolysis has not been demonstrated conclusively in those patients given very early (pre-hospital) thrombolysis.

Non-STEMI presentations

While the NSF and other guidelines have tended to focus on the MI patient with persistent ST segment elevation, there is a growing awareness of the high mortality associated with other presentations of ACS, mandating a more aggressive approach with both medication and PCI. The key to directing appropriate treatment rests with careful risk stratification during the acute presentation.

Summary

The management of the patient with suspected ACS (or 'heart attack') is continually evolving in response to increased knowledge of the pathophysiology and the introduction of new treatments. Policy initiatives have resulted in improved performance in emergency cardiac care, but there remains a need for continuous and sustained effort to reduce treatment delays and improve access to evidence-based treatment.

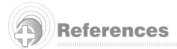
References

Alpert KA, Thygesen K, Antman E et al 2000 Myocardial infarction redefined – a consensus document of The Joint European Society of Cardiology/American College of Cardiology Committee for the redefinition of myocardial infarction. Journal of the American College of Cardiology 36:959–969

Antman E, Anbe DT, Armstrong PW et al 2004 ACC/AHA guidelines for the management of patients with ST-elevation myocardial infarction; a report of the American College of Cardiology/American Heart Association Task Force on Practice Guidelines (Committee to revise the 1999 guidelines for the management of patients with acute myocardial infarction). Journal of the American College of Cardiology 44:E1–E211

Boersma E, Maas AC, Deckers JW et al 1996 Early thrombolytic treatment in acute myocardial infarction: reappraisal of the golden hour. Lancet 348:771–775

British Heart Foundation 2004 Coronary heart disease statistics database. London: British Heart Foundation. Available: www.heartstats.org 21 February 2005

Department of Health 2000 National service framework for coronary heart disease. Department of Health, London

Fox KA 2004 Management of acute coronary syndromes: an update. Heart 90:698–706

Fox KA, Birkhead J, Wilcox R et al 2004 British Cardiac Society Working Group on the definition of myocardial infarction. Heart 90:603–609

Goodacre S, Cross E, Arnold J et al 2005 The health care burden of acute chest pain. Heart 91:229–230

Ioannidis JP, Salem D, Chew PW et al 2001 Accuracy and clinical effectiveness of out-of-hospital electrocardiography in the diagnosis of acute cardiac ischemia: a meta-analysis. Annals of Emergency Medicine 37:461–470

Kainth A, Hewitt A, Sowden A et al 2004 Systematic review of interventions to reduce delay in patients with suspected heart attack. Emergency Medicine Journal 21:506–508

Keeley E, Boura J, Grines C 2003 Primary angioplasty versus intravenous thrombolytic therapy for acute myocardial infarction: a quantitative review of 23 randomised trials. Lancet 361:13–20

Keeling P, Hughes D, Price L 2003 Safety and feasibility of prehospital thrombolysis carried out by paramedics. British Medical Journal 327: 27–28

Machecourt J, Bonnefoy E, Vanzetto G et al 2005 Primary angioplasty is cost minimizing compared with pre-hospital thrombolysis for patients within 60 min of a percutaneous coronary intervention center: the Comparison of Angioplasty and Pre-hospital Thrombolysis in Acute Myocardial Infarction (CAPTIM) cost-efficacy sub-study. Journal of the American College of Cardiology 45:515–524

Morrison LJ, Verbeek PR, McDonald AC et al 2000 Mortality and pre-hospital thrombolysis for acute myocardial infarction – a meta analysis. Journal of the American Medical Association 283:2686–2692

National Assembly for Wales 2001 Tackling CHD in Wales: implementing through evidence. Welsh Assembly, Cardiff

National Heart Attack Alert Program 1994 Emergency department: rapid identification and treatment of patients with acute myocardial infarction. National Heart Attack Alert Program Coordinating Committee, 60 Minutes to Treatment Working Group. Annals of Emergency Medicine 23:311–329

Norris RM 1998 Fatality outside hospital from acute coronary events in three British health districts, 1994–5. United Kingdom Heart Attack Study Collaborative Group. British Medical Journal 316:1065–1070

Pedley DK, Bisset K, Connolly EM et al 2003 Prospective observational cohort study of time saved by prehospital thrombolysis for ST elevation myocardial infarction delivered by paramedics. British Medical Journal 327:22–26

Quinn T, Thompson DR 1995 Administration of thrombolytic therapy to patients with acute myocardial infarction. Accident and Emergency Nursing 3:208–214

Quinn T, Butters A, Todd I 2002 Implementing paramedic thrombolysis – an overview. Accident and Emergency Nursing 10:189–196

Scottish Executive 2002 Coronary heart disease and stroke strategy for Scotland. The Stationery Office, Edinburgh

Silber S, Albertsson P, Aviles F et al 2005 The Task Force for Percutaneous Coronary Interventions of the European Society of Cardiology: guidelines for percutaneous coronary interventions. European Heart Journal 26:804–847

Van de Werf F, Ardissino D, Betriu A et al 2003 The Task Force on the Management of Acute Myocardial Infarction of the European Society of Cardiology: Management of acute myocardial infarction in patients presenting with ST-segment elevation. European Heart Journal 24:28–66

Woollard M, Pitt K, Hayward A et al 2005 Limited benefits of ambulance telemetry in delivering early thrombolysis: a randomised controlled trial. Emergency Medicine Journal 22:209–215

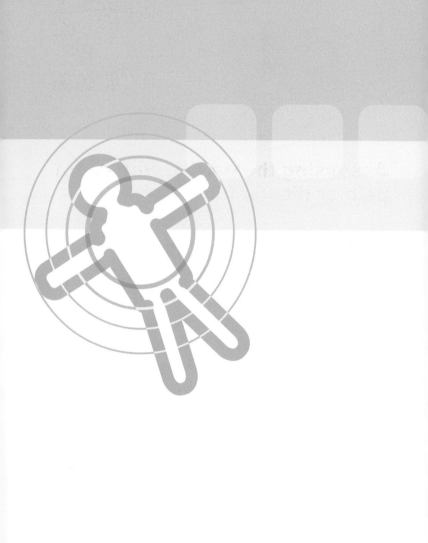

Chapter 2

Assessing the patient with chest pain or discomfort

Chapter contents

Introduction	18
Location	19
Radiation	20
Character	20
Exacerbating or relieving factors	21
Duration and frequency	21
Associated symptoms	21
Atypical presentations	22

This chapter:

- describes the common presentations and diagnosis of ACS

- discusses atypical presentations

- outlines other causes of chest pain.

Introduction

Healthcare staff play key roles in the initial management of patients with suspected ACS: responding rapidly to patients and providing very early access to defibrillation; helping to correctly identify ACS and initiating early triage and treatment including pain relief, aspirin and reperfusion treatments where appropriate. Birkhead et al (2004) report that most decisions to initiate thrombolytic or other reperfusion treatment are made by emergency department doctors, although increasingly such decisions are being made by nurses and paramedics.

Speed is of the essence during the initial patient assessment. History taking should be brief and focused on the identification of the reperfusion-eligible patient. This applies whether thrombolytics or PCI are in local use. A complete clerking is unnecessary at this stage and can lead to dangerous delays in starting treatment. Every effort should be made (e.g. through standardised care pathways and documentation) to avoid unnecessary duplication of assessment. The key questions to be considered are shown in Box 2.1.

Despite the availability of several biochemical markers of myocardial necrosis, the clinical history and ECG are the key factors in determining eligibility for reperfusion treatments. In assessing patients with chest pain some prompts can help

BOX: **2.1** 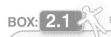 |||||||||||||||||||||||||||||||||||||||||||||||||||||||||||||||||||

Key questions in patient assessment

- Do the presenting symptoms suggest ACS?
- If yes, is there 12-lead ECG evidence of STEMI or LBBB?
- What is the duration of major symptoms?
- If the patient fits the clinical picture of ACS and has STEMI or LBBB and is within the necessary time window, are there any contraindications to thrombolysis and aspirin? Is primary angioplasty indicated and available as a timely alternative?

BOX: **2.2** 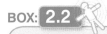 |||||||||||||||||||||||||||||||||||||||||||||||||||||||||||||||||||||||||

Prompts to establish the cause of symptoms

- Location of pain or discomfort
- Radiation
- Character
- Exacerbating or relieving factors
- Duration
- Frequency
- Associated symptoms

establish the cause of symptoms (Box 2.2). These are discussed in more detail below.

Location

A working diagnosis of ACS is typically based upon a history of severe central chest pain lasting for 20 min or more and unrelieved by glyceryl trinitrate (GTN). The patient would not normally be able to isolate the pain by pointing to it with a finger (Braunwald 1997, Jowett & Thompson 2004).

Radiation

It is common for chest pain or discomfort associated with ACS to radiate to – or even be isolated in – one or both arms, the neck, jaw, shoulders, back or even the teeth. Right-sided radiation of chest pain, while uncommon, has a high 'likelihood ratio' for MI (Mant et al 2004). There is some evidence of gender differences in symptom presentation associated with MI, with women more likely than men to describe pain in the back, neck or jaw (Goldberg et al 1998).

Character

Common descriptors for the pain associated with ACS include:

- 'crushing'
- 'vice-like constriction'
- 'heartburn'
- or like something 'sitting on the chest' (Antman et al 2004).

Pain severity is often assessed using a numerical rating scale of 0 or 1 (pain absent) to 10 (worst pain). Not all patients with ACS describe 'chest pain' but may complain instead of 'discomfort'. Beware the middle-aged man with 'indigestion', particularly if there is no previous history of dyspepsia (Moulten & Yates 1999).

Patients who have pre-existing CHD may be able to make useful comparisons to previous episodes; for example 'worse than my normal angina' or 'like the last time I had a heart attack'. Patients' actual experience of heart attack often differs from pre-conceived ideas of a 'sudden dramatic event in which people collapse and die' (Ruston et al 1998).

Mant et al (2004) found that the clinical features most helpful in ruling *out* the diagnosis of ACS were the presence of pleuritic, sharp or positional pain and pain produced by palpation.

Exacerbating or relieving factors

The pain associated with ACS is not normally worse on inspiration nor made worse by coughing. Positional pain and pain produced by palpation are less likely to be due to ACS, as discussed above. If the patient has a history of exertional symptoms relieved by resting, this would suggest the presence of myocardial ischaemia. Pain due to ACS, however, typically occurs at rest.

Duration and frequency

The pain associated with ACS typically lasts for at least 20–30 min, though the severity may vary over this period. A proportion of patients who present with ACS – even though they have not been previously diagnosed with angina – will have had a recent history of non-specific chest pain. This phenomenon may actually help to protect the heart by a process called 'preconditioning' (Ishihara et al 1997).

Associated symptoms

The pain or discomfort of ACS is frequently associated with shortness of breath, diaphoresis (sweating), weakness, nausea and vomiting, and sometimes with belching and 'indigestion' (see above). Such symptoms can cause diagnostic difficulties. Goldberg et al (1998) found that women were more likely to experience nausea whilst men were more likely to report diaphoresis.

Observation of non-verbal cues can also be useful when assessing a patient's pain. For example, clenching the fist in front of the sternum (Levine's sign) may be an indication that the pain is of ischaemic origin (Braunwald 1997).

Atypical presentations

Patients can present with atypical symptoms. Clinical suspicion of ACS in the absence of 'classic' symptoms should be taken seriously and further investigations are warranted. Chest pain observation units have been developed to help meet the needs of patients with this phenomenon (Herren and Mackway-Jones 2001).

'Silent' myocardial ischaemia is a well-recognised phenomenon (Wong & White 2002) and accounts for 20% of all patients with a final diagnosis of MI (Dorsch et al 2001). Brieger et al (2004) found that patients who presented atypically were likely to be older, female, hypertensive, diabetic and to have had a history of heart failure. Atypical features are more likely to be present in patients from certain minority ethnic groups (Barakat et al 2003). Although all patients with painless ACS should be treated according to standard guidelines, diagnosis is often delayed and treatment suboptimal (Brieger et al 2004). Whether or not to administer thrombolysis to a patient with STEMI but no chest discomfort can, in practice, be a difficult decision because of uncertainty in determining the time of onset (Wong & White 2002), but

Table 2.1 Non-ACS causes of chest pain

Life threatening causes	Non-ACS cardiac causes	Non-cardiac causes
Aortic dissection	Pericarditis	Gastric reflux
Pulmonary embolism	Myocarditis	Pleuritic pain
Perforated ulcer	Hypertrophic cardiomyopathy	Chest wall syndrome
Tension pneumothorax		Peptic ulceration
Oesophageal rupture		Panic attacks
		Hepatobiliary disease
		Cervical pathology
		Psychogenic causes

many senior clinicians would advocate the administration of the treatment where there is persistent ST segment elevation. Primary PCI may be a preferred alternative if locally available.

Beware patients with atypical presentations. This group has a higher mortality associated, in part, with lower use of effective treatments.

ACS is not the only cause of chest discomfort

There are many non-ACS causes of chest pain, some of which require immediate treatment (e.g. acute aortic dissection, pulmonary embolism). These are shown in Table 2.1, although the list is not exhaustive.

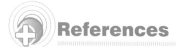 **References**

Antman EM, Anbe DT, Armstrong PW et al 2004 ACC/AHA guidelines for the management of patients with ST-elevation myocardial infarction; a report of the American College of Cardiology/American Heart Association Task Force on Practice Guidelines (Committee to revise the 1999 guidelines for the management of patients with acute myocardial infarction). Journal of the American College of Cardiology 44:E1–E211

Barakat K, Wells Z, Ramdhany S et al 2003 Bangladeshi patients present with non-classic features of acute myocardial infarction and are treated less aggressively in east London, UK. Heart 89:276–279

Birkhead JS, Walker L, Pearson M et al 2004 on behalf of the MINAP Steering Group. Improving care for patients with acute coronary syndromes: initial results from the National Audit of Myocardial Infarction Project (MINAP). Heart 90:1004–1009

Braunwald E 1997 The history. In: Braunwald E (ed.) Heart disease: a textbook of cardiovascular medicine: Part 1 Examination of the patient, 5th edn. WB Saunders, Philadelphia, p 1–14

Brieger D, Eagle KA, Goodman SG et al 2004 Acute coronary syndromes without chest pain, an underdiagnosed and undertreated high-risk group: insights from the Global Registry of Acute Coronary Events. Chest 126:461–469

Dorsch M, Lawrance R, Sapsford R et al 2001 for the EMMACE Study Group. Poor prognosis of patients presenting with symptomatic myocardial infarction but without chest pain. Heart 86:494–498

Goldberg RJ, O'Donnell C, Yarzebski J et al 1998 Sex differences in symptom presentation associated with acute myocardial infarction: a population-based perspective. American Heart Journal 136:189–195

Herren KR, Mackway-Jones K 2001 Emergency management of cardiac chest pain: a review. Emergency Medical Journal 18:6–10

Ishihara M, Sato H, Tateishi H et al 1997 Implications of prodromal angina pectoris in anterior wall acute myocardial infarction: acute angiographic findings and long-term prognosis. Journal of the American College of Cardiology 30:970–975

Jowett NI, Thompson DR 2003 Comprehensive coronary care, 3rd edn. Baillière Tindall, London, p 67

Mant J, McManus RJ, Oakes RAL et al 2004 Systematic review and modelling of the investigation of acute chest pain presenting in primary care. Health Technology Assessment 8:1–158

Moulten C, Yates D 1999 Lecture notes on emergency medicine, 2nd edn. Blackwell Science, Oxford, p 161

Ruston A, Clayton J, Calnan M 1998 Patients' action during their cardiac event: qualitative study exploring differences and modifiable factors. British Medical Journal 316:1060–1064

Wong CK, White HD 2002 Recognising 'painless' heart attacks. Heart 87:3–5

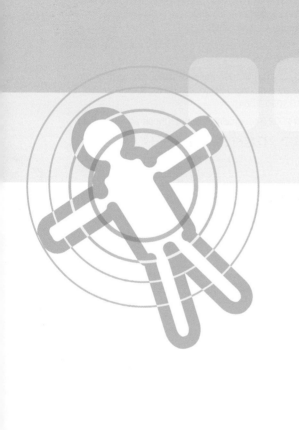

Chapter 3

Immediate management

Chapter contents

Immediate priorities   28

Assessing vital signs   29

Aspirin and clopidogrel   29

Oxygen   30

Nitrates   30

Recording the 12-lead ECG   30

Establishing intravenous access   31

Administering pain relief   31

This chapter:

- discusses the immediate priorities of care for patients with suspected ACS, whether initially seen by paramedics, other primary care professionals or hospital clinicians.

Immediate priorities

As discussed in the previous chapter, chest pain is the most common symptom associated with ACS and there needs to be a high index of suspicion that any chest pain is cardiac in origin. Patients with ACS who do *not* present with chest pain as the chief complaint, but who have related symptoms such as dyspnoea and sweating, are an important group at high risk of death and other complications.

Initial assessment should be as rapid and focused as possible. Early care focuses on resuscitation where required (see inside front cover), pain relief, establishing a working diagnosis and initiating appropriate treatment. Both patients and their loved ones are likely to be highly anxious and a calm, caring approach that balances the need to safeguard dignity while maintaining patient safety is required. Initial priorities of care include:

- Assessing vital signs: Airway, Breathing, Circulation (a defibrillator should be immediately available). For treatment of cardiac arrest, see inside front cover. For treatment of arrhythmias, see Chapter 7.

- Administering 300 mg aspirin (if no contraindications and not already given)

- Giving supplementary oxygen (initially high flow, but exercise caution in chronic obstructive pulmonary disease (COPD))

- Giving nitrates (sublingual or buccal) to attempt to ease discomfort (unless contraindicated, see p. 30, 144)

- Recording a good quality 12-lead ECG and identifying changes requiring immediate action, such as reperfusion treatments
- Establishing intravenous (IV) access
- Administering adequate (usually opiate) pain relief with an anti-emetic (see below)
- Assessment for reperfusion (discussed in Chapters 8 and 10).

Allow the patient to sit or lie in whatever position is most comfortable (most patients with ischaemic chest pain will prefer to sit up).

Reassurance of the patient is vital: anxiety is a natural and understandable response to a suspected 'heart attack'.

Assessing vital signs

The heart rate and blood pressure should be monitored continually, with the patient attached to an ECG monitor if available. Pulse oximetry also provides useful information.

Aspirin and clopidogrel

Aspirin has been shown to reduce mortality and adverse events in patients with acute myocardial infarction (AMI) and unstable angina. In the ISIS II (1988) trial, aspirin alone was shown to save almost as many lives as streptokinase alone following AMI. 300 mg should be given, chewed or dispersed in water, provided there are no contraindications (true contraindications to this lifesaving drug are rare). Patients who are truly aspirin intolerant may benefit from administration of clopidogrel. Whilst evidence is emerging which suggests clopidogrel may have a role in the management of STEMI, in addition to aspirin,

at the time of writing this is not established practice. Both drugs
are used in NSTEMI and unstable angina.

Oxygen

Oxygen is recommended routinely for patients with suspected
ACS, particularly in the early phase of care and in those who
have complications, such as ongoing pain, arrhythmia, shock
or heart failure. The evidence base for supplementary oxygen
administration in uncomplicated patients is weak (Nicholson
2004). Care should be exercised in patients with chronic
pulmonary disease.

Nitrates

Nitrates are effective at providing symptomatic relief in stable
angina. Although not shown to improve outcomes following
MI, nitrates are useful in the immediate care of an ACS patient
in reducing symptoms, principally through vasodilation.

Nitrates can cause headaches and patients should be warned
of this. The risks of hypotension are increased in patients
receiving concurrent opiate treatment. Nitrates should not be
administered to patients with a systolic blood pressure less than
90 mmHg (or greater than or equal to 30 mmHg below the
patient's baseline), bradycardia, tachycardia or suspected right-
ventricular infarction (Antman et al 2004).

Recording the 12-lead ECG

A good quality 12-lead ECG is essential in the early assessment
of the patient with suspected ACS. Taking a 12-lead ECG is
covered in detail in Chapter 4.

Establishing intravenous access

Use of the IV route for injections is mandatory in the immediate care of patients with suspected ACS: opiate analgesia and other parenterally administered medicines are likely to be more readily (and predictably) absorbed and the risk of haematoma accompanying use of thrombolytic, antiplatelet and related treatments is reduced. Moreover, intramuscular injections can result in biomarker rise, which can interfere with the diagnostic process. Exceptions to this rule include subcutaneous administration of low-molecular-weight heparin (LMWH) and insulin where required. The IV route is also required for administration of medication to treat rhythm disturbances and in the event of cardiac arrest.

Administering pain relief

Pain relief should be given as a matter of urgency both for humanitarian reasons and also to reduce the risk of adverse events associated with catecholamine release.

The opiate of choice in prehospital care is morphine: 5–10 mg by slow IV injection (2 mg/min) titrated to response. A further 5–10 mg may be given if necessary. The dose may need to be reduced in elderly or frail patients (BNF 2005). Alternatively, diamorphine can be given: 2.5–5 mg by slow IV injection (1 mg/min) followed by a further 2.5–5 mg if necessary. Again, the dose may need to be reduced in elderly or frail patients (BNF 2005).

Opiates are routinely accompanied by an anti-emetic, typically metoclopramide 10 mg IV. Cyclizine and prochlorperazine should be avoided.

Reversal of respiratory depression induced by opiates is occasionally required, using naloxone 100–200 µg

(1.5–3 μg/kg), IV. The dose can be repeated every 2 min to
achieve the desired effect. Atropine should be readily available
in the event of opiate-induced bradycardia (Antman et al
2004).

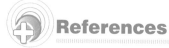

References

Antman EM, Anbe DT, Armstrong PW et al 2004 ACC/AHA guidelines
for the management of patients with ST-elevation myocardial infarction;
A report of the American College of Cardiology/American Heart
Association Task Force on Practice Guidelines (Committee to revise the
1999 guidelines for the management of patients with acute myocardial
infarction). Journal of the American College of Cardiology 44:E1–E211

BNF 2005 British National Formulary 49. British Medical Association & Royal
Pharmaceutical Society of Great Britain, London

ISIS–2. (Second international study of infarct survival) Collaborative
Group 1988 Randomised trial of intravenous streptokinase, oral aspirin,
both or neither among 17187 cases of suspected acute myocardial
infarction. Lancet 2:349–360

Nicholson C 2004 A systematic review of the effectiveness of oxygen in
reducing acute myocardial ischaemia. Journal of Clinical Nursing
13:996–1007

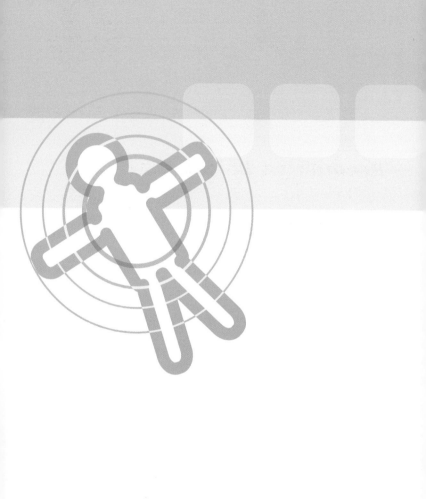

Recording a 12-lead ECG

Chapter contents

Introduction	36
The 12-lead ECG	37
Ensuring a high quality ECG recording	37
Electrode placement	38
Right-sided and posterior ECG leads	40

This chapter:

- discusses the importance of the ECG as a diagnostic tool in suspected ACS

- outlines the key principles related to recording a12-lead ECG.

Introduction

When assessing a patient with suspected ACS, the 12-lead ECG forms the cornerstone of decision making. It should be recorded at the first opportunity either by ambulance personnel or, if the patient self-presents to a hospital or primary care setting, by appropriately trained staff. Decisions about reperfusion using thrombolytics or referral for primary PCI are made largely on the basis of ECG findings combined with clinical history. Very rarely (if ever) are such decisions made on biochemical marker release.

The ECG needs to be interpreted by a suitably experienced clinician immediately. In the ambulance setting this may be by paramedics or it may be facilitated remotely by hospital or ambulance personnel via telemetry or fax transmission.

For safety reasons it is important to ensure that the patient's name appears on the ECG. An ECG without a name on it poses a potential risk to the patient and should not be used for making treatment decisions.

If the initial ECG is non-diagnostic of STEMI but the patient remains symptomatic and there is a high index of suspicion, repeat recordings at frequent intervals (every 5–10 min as a minimum). Continuous ST segment monitoring may be helpful if available.

The 12-lead ECG

The 12-lead ECG is of prime importance in the assessment of the patient with suspected ACS. Whilst it is possible to gain limited information from a single ECG lead – such as that produced by a cardiac monitor or defibrillator paddles – a 12-lead ECG provides much more information.

In the context of cardiac-sounding symptoms, an ECG showing ST elevation is a key finding that necessitates immediate action. Other significant findings are bundle branch block (BBB) and ST depression, which also identify patients at high risk of death (Fibrinolytic Therapy Trialists' Collaborative Group 1994). All ECGs must be interpreted within the clinical context.

A normal ECG does not exclude ACS!

Ensuring a high-quality ECG recording

When assessing for suspected ACS, the ECG is unlikely to be recorded on a calm, relaxed patient lying comfortably on a bed. Nevertheless, there are some simple measures that can help to optimise the quality of the ECG recording:

- The practitioner should have a calm, confident manner

- The procedure should be explained to the patient; emphasising that it is painless and is used only for recording the heart's electrical activity

- The patient should be made as comfortable as is possible in the circumstances. All limbs should be on a supportive surface as this will help to minimise interference due to muscle tremor

- The skin over the electrode site on the limbs and chest should be clean and dry prior to electrode application

- Leathery, suntanned or dry skin should be gently abraded, if possible, to reduce impedance (electrical resistance between the patient and the ECG machine).

- Chest hair should be carefully shaved, if necessary

- The identification information on the ECG should accurately match the patient's details.

Electrode placement

As 12-lead ECGs are often recorded sequentially for comparison and interpretation, parameters are based on longstanding international convention; it is important that precordial (chest) leads are recorded from the same position each time an ECG is taken (see below).

Self-adhesive electrodes are now in almost universal use. The operator should consider:

- applying all electrodes before connecting to the ECG machine as this 'time on skin' may enhance adhesion and also reduce impedance

- avoiding strain on the lead wires, when attaching the electrodes, by pointing the electrode tabs towards the patient's abdomen, in the direction of lead wire 'pull'.

Limb electrodes

The limb electrodes are placed as shown in Figure 4.1.

The chest electrodes

The chest electrodes are placed as follows (Fig. 4.2):

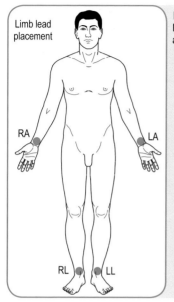

Limb lead placement

RA

LA

RL   LL

Figure 4.1 Limb lead placement. RA: right arm; RL: right leg; LA: left arm; LL: left leg.

- V1 4th intercostal space to the right of the sternum
- V2 4th intercostal space to the left of the sternum
- V3 directly between V2 and V4
- V4 5th intercostal space, midclavicular line
- V5 level with V4 on the left anterior axillary line
- V6 level with V5 on the midaxillary line (midpoint of the axilla).

Breast tissue appears to have little effect on ECG amplitude and, in women, the placement of chest electrodes over, rather than under, the breast has been recommended by some authors (Rautaharju et al 1998). Either approach seems to make little difference, if any, to subsequent decision making, but deviation

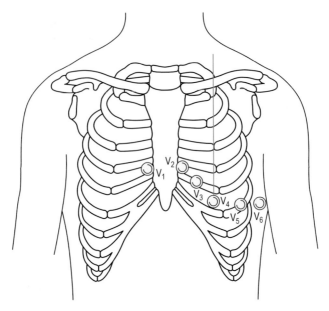

Figure 4.2 Electrode positions of the precordial leads.
Reproduced with permission from Thompson & Webster (2005).

from 'conventional' electrode placement positions should
always be documented.

Right-sided and posterior ECG leads

While the trial evidence for the benefits of thrombolytic
treatment has been derived from conventional 12-lead ECG
data, useful information may be obtained from recordings of
additional leads. In the hospital setting, patients who present
with ECG evidence of inferior STEMI should also have right-
sided ECG leads recorded to exclude right ventricular infarction

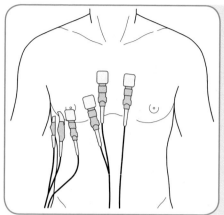

Figure 4.3 Right-sided electrode placement.

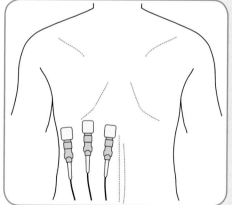

Figure 4.4 Posterior electrode placement.

(Fig. 4.3) (Carley 2003, Antman et al 2004). This and other additional lead recording is less convenient in the ambulance setting but is likely to become more popular in the future, possibly in association with emerging techniques such as body surface mapping (Carley et al 2005).

If posterior infarction is suspected (e.g. in the context of ST elevation in inferior leads and presence of positive R wave in V1 and associated ST depression, as discussed in Chapter 5) it may be useful to obtain leads V7–V9 (Brady & Morris 1999, Matetzky et al 1998). These leads are placed in the same intercostal space as V4–V6, but continue 'round the back' of the patient as shown in Figure 4.4. The appropriate leads should be marked V7–V9 on the ECG.

 References

Antman EM, Anbe DT, Armstrong PW et al 2004 ACC/AHA guidelines for the management of patients with ST-elevation myocardial infarction; A report of the American College of Cardiology/American Heart Association Task Force on Practice Guidelines (Committee to revise the 1999 guidelines for the management of patients with acute myocardial infarction). Journal of the American College of Cardiology 44:E1–E211

Brady JW, Morris F 1999 The additional lead electrocardiogram in acute myocardial infarction. Journal of Accident and Emergency Medicine 16:202–207

Carley SD 2003 Beyond the 12 lead: review of the use of additional leads for the early electrocardiographic diagnosis of acute myocardial infarction. Emergency Medicine 15:143–154

Carley SD, Jenkins M, Jones KM 2005 Body surface mapping versus the standard 12 lead ECG in the detection of myocardial infarction amongst emergency department patients: a Bayesian approach. Resuscitation 64:309–314

Fibrinolytic Therapy Trialists' (FTT) Collaborative Group 1994 Indications for fibrinolytic therapy in suspected acute myocardial infarction: collaborative overview of early mortality and major morbidity results from all randomised trials of more than 1000 patients. Lancet 343: 311–322

Matetzky S, Freimark D, Chouraqui P et al 1998 Significance of ST segment elevations in posterior chest leads (V7 to V9) in patients with acute inferior myocardial infarction: application for thrombolytic therapy. Journal of the American College of Cardiology 31:506–511

Rautaharju PM, Park L, Rautaharju FS et al 1998 A standardized procedure for locating and documenting ECG chest electrode positions: consideration of the effect of breast tissue on ECG amplitudes in women. Journal of Electrocardiology 31:17–29

Thompson DR, Webster RA 2005 Caring for the coronary patient, 2nd edn. Butterworth-Heinemann, London

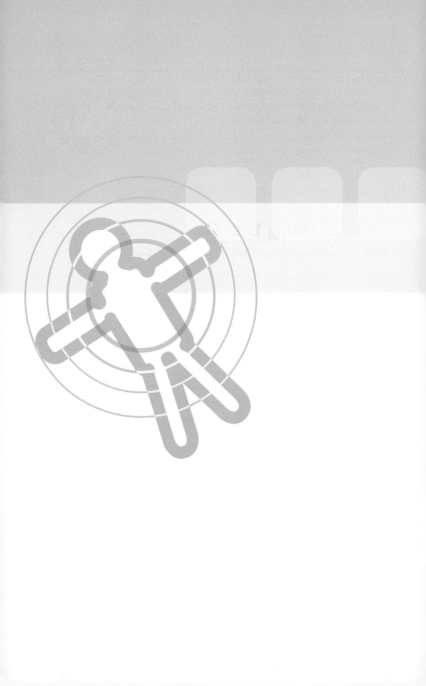

Chapter 5

Interpreting the 12-lead ECG in the patient with suspected ACS

Chapter contents

Introduction   46

The ST segment   47

ECG orientation   50

STEMI   51

Bundle branch block   58

Other causes of ST elevation   59

Non-ST elevation ACS   60

This chapter:

- discusses the principles that underpin the interpretation of a 12-lead ECG in the context of suspected ACS

- relates those principles to identifying specific areas of the 'at risk' myocardium with an emphasis on ST segment elevation and ST segment depression, with additional reference to bundle branch block.

Introduction

The main acute ECG manifestations of ACS are:

- ST elevation MI (STEMI)

- Non-ST elevation MI (NSTEMI) (characterised principally by ST depression)

- Bundle branch block (BBB).

There should be systems in place to ensure that all patients being assessed for suspected ACS have a 12-lead ECG taken without delay. A competent member of staff should review the ECG.

If the first ECG is inconclusive but the patient's symptoms are suspicious then the recording should be repeated at regular intervals.

Distinguishing between the above manifestations on the ECG is important because thrombolytic treatment has only been proven to be of benefit in patients with STEMI or BBB (mainly left BBB). The benefits of thrombolysis by presenting ECG category are summarised in Table 5.1.

Box 5.1 shows the criteria for the diagnosis of STEMI.

Table 5.1 35-day mortality in relation to entry ECG (Reprinted from FTT Collaborative Group 1994)

ECG	Mortality with thrombolysis	Mortality with placebo
ST elevation anterior	13.2	16.9
ST elevation inferior	7.5	8.4
ST depression	15.2	13.8
Bundle branch block	18.7	23.6
Normal	3	2.3

BOX: **5.1** 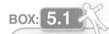 ||||||||||||||||||||||||||||||||||||||||||||||||||||||||||||||||||||||||

Commonly used ECG criteria for reperfusion

1. 1mm ST elevation (or more) in 2 or more contiguous (adjacent) <u>limb</u> leads.
   or
2. 2mm ST elevation (or more) in 2 contiguous <u>chest</u> leads (V1–V6).
   or
3. (presumed new) LBBB.

The ST segment

The QRS represents electrical depolarisation of the ventricles (leading to ventricular contraction). The T wave signifies the resting (repolarisation) phase of the heart. The *ST segment* is

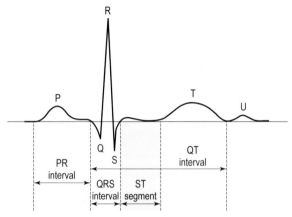

Figure 5.1 ECG complex with ST segment highlighted.

situated between the QRS and the T wave. More specifically, it starts at the 'J point' – the junction of the S wave and the ST segment (see Fig. 5.1) and ends at the start of the T wave (in acute MI the start of the T wave may not be visible).

On a normal ECG the ST segment is curved very slightly upwards, but is usually isoelectric; that is, it originates from the baseline. Thrombolysis eligibility criteria tend to allow for some normal variation in the ST segments.

The significance of the ST segment lies in its sensitivity to myocardial injury. For example, in a 'classic' MI – a STEMI – the ST segment rises above the baseline, a finding that is vital when making decisions about reperfusion therapy (FTT 1994).

The amount of ST elevation is determined by measuring the height of the ST segment compared to the baseline. In STEMI, the ST segment tends to lose its upwardly concave shape and becomes straightened with an upward slope. This straight upward slope then becomes elevated (Schamroth 1990).

A normal ST segment

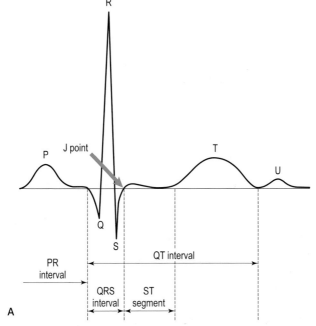

Figure 5.2A & B These diagrams show J point in normal ECG complex and in the presence of ST elevation. Note: some practitioners use the J point to determine the amount of ST elevation whilst others use alternative points of reference; for example 80 ms past the J point; refer to local practice.

In practice, the reference point for ST elevation measurement seems to vary depending on who is measuring it (Carley et al 2002). For example, some practitioners use the J point, whilst others may use J point + 80 ms (2 small squares horizontally) (Fig. 5.2). Furthermore, there seems to be a lack of consensus in the literature on the best point of measurement, though some texts do refer to the J point in this context. However, when ST changes are obvious, such subtleties are irrelevant.

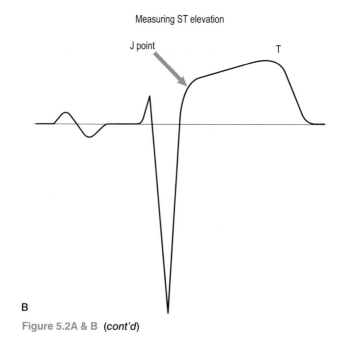

Measuring ST elevation

B

Figure 5.2A & B (*cont'd*)

ECG orientation

Figure 5.3 shows the layout of the 12 leads on an ECG produced by a modern electrocardiograph. Often, as here, there will be a rhythm strip running the length of the lower part of the page. By convention, the left half of the display shows the limb leads, while the right half shows chest leads V1–V6.

The ECG can help to determine which part of the heart is affected by ischaemia, injury or infarction, and can also identify other abnormalities. The remainder of this chapter

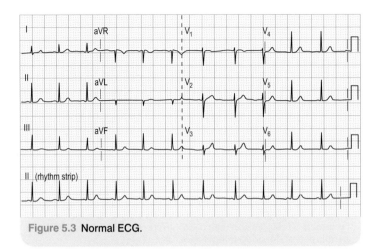

Figure 5.3 Normal ECG.

will concentrate on ECG changes associated with the ACS patient.

STEMI

Inferior MI

Figure 5.4 shows the site of injury in inferior MI.

Leads II, III, and aVF are orientated to the inferior part of the left ventricle. ST elevation in these leads is therefore indicative of an inferior MI. ST segment changes in these leads are usually associated with right coronary artery (RCA) obstruction. An inferior STEMI can be complicated by bradycardia because the RCA frequently also provides the blood supply to the SA and AV node.

Note: A diagnosis of STEMI is made in the presence of ST elevation in any two of the three leads II, III and aVF.

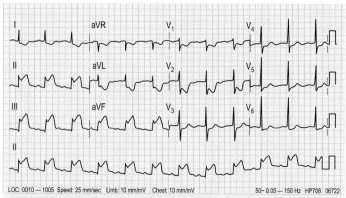

Figure 5.4 Inferior MI; marked ST elevation in II, III, aVF and reciprocal ST depression (see p. 55). (Reproduced with the kind permission of Boehringer Ingelheim, UK.)

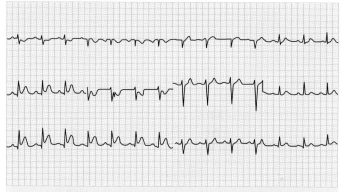

Figure 5.5 ECG showing ST elevation in II, III, and aVF, denoting acute inferior MI.

Further examples of 12-lead ECGs showing inferior MI

The ECG shown in Figure 5.5 shows ST segment elevation indicative of acute inferior MI. Figure 5.6 shows more subtle changes in ST elevation in two leads, but still indicates inferior MI.

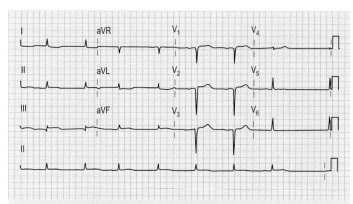

Figure 5.6 ECG showing more subtle changes (1mm) ST elevation in leads III and aVF. Note the bradycardia.

Right ventricular infarction (RVI) involvement in inferior STEMI

Due to the occlusion of the RCA, right ventricular infarction (RVI) occurs in approximately 20–30% of patients with inferior STEMI. This has important implications for the management of patients if hypotension or shock develops (see Chapter 6). It is therefore considered good practice in hospitals routinely to record right ventricular leads in patients with inferior STEMI (see Fig. 4.3 for details of electrode placement), although the value of recording these additional leads in the ambulance setting is unknown. Lead V4R is considered to be of particular value diagnostically.

Figure 5.7 shows an ECG recording of right ventricular leads RV3–RV6 indicating RVI involvement.

Anterior MI

Figure 5.8 shows the site of injury in anterior MI in relation to the 12-lead ECG.

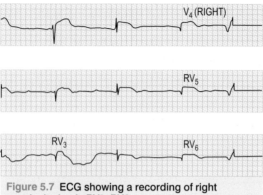

Figure 5.7 ECG showing a recording of right ventricular leads RV3–RV6.

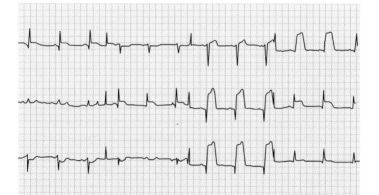

Figure 5.8 ECG showing ST elevation in V1–V6 denoting extensive anterior MI. (Reproduced with the kind permission of Boehringer Ingelheim, UK.)

LeadsV1–V6 look at the front surface of the left ventricle. It is these leads that are affected during an anterior MI.

Leads V1–V6 cover a relatively large area of myocardium so terms such as 'anterolateral' tend to be used to denote the exact area affected. Specific terminology will vary though. As a general rule:

- ST elevation in V2–V6 is referred to as an *anterior MI*
- ST elevation in I, aVL, V2–V6 is referred to as an *anterolateral MI*
- ST elevation in V5 and V6 is referred to as a *lateral (or apical) MI.*

The key priority is to identify ST elevation and to make a decision regarding reperfusion eligibility, whether by pharmacological (thrombolysis) or mechanical (PCI) means.

An anterior STEMI is usually associated with occlusion of the left coronary artery. The large area of myocardium supplied by this major vessel means that there is high risk of heart failure and shock in the absence of timely reperfusion.

Note: in both anterior and inferior MI, ST elevation in some leads can be accompanied by ST depression in others and this is associated with increased risk of complications, including death. The term *'reciprocal ST depression'* is sometimes used to describe this.

Posterior MI

Acute posterior wall MI occurs in up to 20% of MI patients, though it is usually a secondary finding in the context of inferior or lateral STEMI (Pollehn et al 2002). In the absence of ST elevation in conventional ECG leads, a suspected true posterior MI can give rise to difficulty in decision making; thrombolysis may be harmful in patients presenting with ST depression alone (FTT 1994). The presence of horizontal ST depression with tall upright T waves in V1, V2 or V3 and/or a tall wide R wave

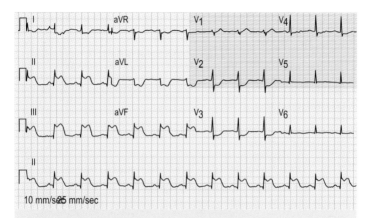

10 mm/s 25 mm/sec

Figure 5.9 ECG showing acute inferior MI with tall R waves and ST segment depression in leads V2 and V3 indicative of possible associated posterior wall involvement. Thrombolysis or primary PCI would be indicated on the basis of the ST elevation in this case.

in those leads may support the diagnosis (Pollehn et al 2002). Where the diagnosis of posterior wall MI is suspected, advice from a senior clinician (e.g. a consultant cardiologist) should be obtained before initiating thrombolytic treatment in the absence of ST elevation.

Additional leads can prove useful (see Chapter 4), but it is sensible to seek the opinion of a senior clinician before administering a thrombolytic. Treatment by PCI, if readily available, may be preferable.

Examples of ECGs showing posterior MI

The ECG in Figure 5.9 shows acute inferior MI with tall R waves and ST segment depression in leads V2 and V3, indicative of possible associated posterior wall involvement. Thrombolysis or primary PCI would be indicated on the basis of the ST elevation in this case.

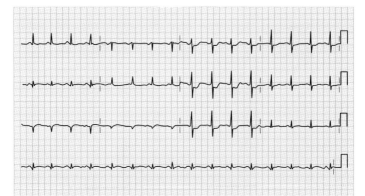

Figure 5.10 ECG showing ST segment depression in V1–V3 without discernible ST elevation in leads II, III & aVF. This could indicate NSTEMI or posterior wall MI.

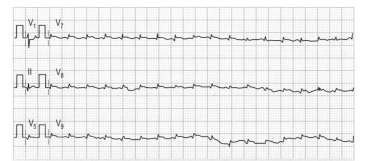

Figure 5.11 ECG recording from the same patient as Figure 5.10. Leads V7–V9 show subtle ST segment elevation suggestive of possible isolated posterior wall MI.

Figure 5.10 shows ST segment depression in V1–V3 without discernible ST elevation in leads II, III and aVF. This could indicate non-STEMI or posterior wall MI. Figure 5.11 shows an ECG recording from leads V7–V9 from the same patient – subtle

Table 5.2 Incidence of ECG findings in context of AMI and their associated mortality (Terkelsen et al 2005).

	Incidence	Mortality at 1 year
Non STEMI	54%	31%
STEMI	39%	21%
BBB	6%	55%

ST segment elevation suggests possible isolated posterior wall MI. Reperfusion (thrombolysis or primary PCI) would normally be indicated: consult a senior clinician.

Bundle branch block (BBB)

BBB is present in around 6% of patients with MI and is associated with a very high mortality (Terkelsen et al 2005), as shown in Table 5.2. As a significant proportion of patients who present with BBB will *not* be experiencing an MI, it is useful to have a previous ECG available, where possible, to help establish whether or not the changes are new. This may be a paper-based or electronic resource (Gamon & Cooper 2002), the latter being facilitated by the wider introduction of electronic patient records.

Figure 5.12 shows a 12-lead ECG showing LBBB.

The presence of right BBB (RBBB) on the ECG is not an indication for thrombolysis in itself (unlike new LBBB) – ST elevation is also required. In the presence of BBB (either left or right), primary PCI may be the preferred reperfusion strategy, if available.

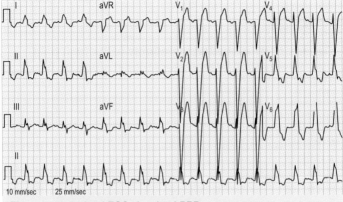

Figure 5.12 12-lead ECG showing LBBB.

Features that may help identify myocardial ischaemia in LBBB (Sgarbossa et al 1996) include:

- ST segment elevation in association with a positive QRS complex, or
- ST segment depression in leads V1, V2 or V3 (termed 'inappropriate concordance' and strongly indicative of ischaemia)
- Profound ST segment elevation in V1 and V2.

Other causes of ST elevation

MI is not the only cause of ST elevation. Brady et al (2001) found that of 202 patients who presented to an A&E department with chest pain and ST elevation, MI was the cause in only 15% of cases (Box 5.2).

BOX: 5.2

Causes of ST elevation in patients with chest pain and ST elevation in an observational study by Brady et al (2001)

- Left ventricular hypertrophy (25%)
- AMI (15%)
- LBBB (15%)
- Benign early repolarisation (12%)
- RBBB(5%)
- Non-specific BBB(5%)
- Left ventricular aneurysm (3%)
- Acute pericarditis (1%)
- Ventricular paced rhythm (1%)
- Undefined ST segment elevation (17%)

If in doubt, obtain a previous ECG and do not delay in seeking the advice of a senior clinician.

Non-ST elevation ACS

Patients with non-ST elevation may present with ST *depression*, such as that shown in Figure 5.13. In such patients, the sum of ST segment depression in all ECG leads is a strong predictor of mortality at 30 days and has been shown to correlate with the extent and severity of coronary artery disease (Savonitto et al 2005). It is important to identify these high risk patients so that appropriate treatment can be commenced and referral for coronary angiography can be made at an early stage (see Chapter 11 for specific management advice). Note that thrombolytic treatment is *not* indicated for these patients.

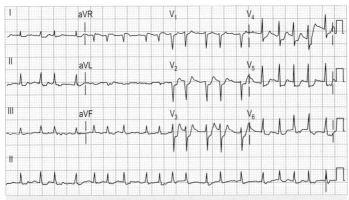

Figure 5.13 ECG showing widespread ST segment depression.

Other ECG changes, such as T wave inversion and left ventricular hypertrophy, also associated with presentations of ACS, indicate patients at high risk. Thrombolysis is not indicated in these groups, but all patients with a clinical suspicion of ACS, irrespective of their presenting ECG, should be risk stratified formally and managed appropriately (see Chapter 11).

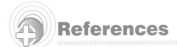 **References**

Brady WJ, Perron AD, Martin ML et al 2001 Cause of ST segment abnormality in ED chest pain patients. American Journal of Emergency Medicine 19:25–28

Carley S, Gamon R, Driscoll P et al 2002 What's the point of ST elevation? Journal of Emergency Medicine 19:126–128

Fibrinolytic Therapy Trialists' (FTT) Collaborative Group 1994 Indications for fibrinolytic therapy in suspected acute myocardial infarction: collaborative overview of early mortality and major morbidity results from all randomised trials of more than 1000 patients. Lancet 343:311–322

Gamon R, Cooper A 2002 Applying an ECG database to aid decision-making in the A&E department. A&E Nursing Journal 10:62–64

Pollehn T, Brady WJ, Perron AD et al 2002 The electrocardiographic differential diagnosis of ST segment depression. Emergency Medical Journal 19:129–135

Savonitto S, Cohen MG, Politi A et al 2005 Extent of ST-segment depression and cardiac events in non-ST-segment elevation acute coronary syndromes. European Heart Journal 26:2106–2113

Sgarbossa EB, Pinski SL, Barbagelata A et al 1996 Electrocardiographic diagnosis of evolving acute myocardial infarction in the presence of left bundle branch block. GUSTO-I (Global Utilization of Streptokinase and Tissue Plasminogen Activator for Occluded Coronary Arteries) Investigators. New England Journal of Medicine 334:481–487.

Shamroth L 1990 An introduction to electrocardiography, 7th edn. Blackwell Scientific, Oxford

Terkelsen CJ, Lassen JF, Norgaard BL et al 2005 Mortality rates in patients with ST-elevation vs. non-ST-elevation acute myocardial infarction: observations from an unselected cohort. European Heart Journal 26:18–26

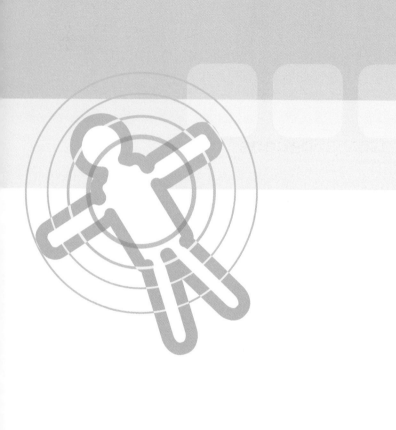

Chapter 6

Complications

Chapter contents

Cardiac arrest	66
Arrhythmias	66
Heart failure	66
Cardiogenic shock	68
Right ventricular infarction	70
Ventricular septal defect/rupture	71

This chapter:

- concentrates particularly on complications of ACS and their treatment

- emphasises that optimal management of complications requires specialist input.

In many of the following circumstances the patient and family members will be highly anxious and distressed. The aim is to provide optimal comfort and support as well as technological intervention.

Cardiac arrest

Refer to the advanced life support and in-hospital resuscitation algorithms on the insides of the front and back covers. Arrhythmias associated with cardiac arrest, and cardiac drugs are discussed in Chapter 7.

Arrhythmias

Arrhythmias are common in patients with ACS. Recognising and managing arrhythmia is discussed in detail in Chapter 7.

Heart failure

Heart failure is a common and serious complication in ACS patients, carrying a poor prognosis. Heart failure is more common in patients with STEMI or LBBB who have delayed (or no) reperfusion treatment. Initial heart rate and blood pressure recordings may give an indication of subsequent risk of death following MI (Das et al 2005).

Auscultation of the heart and lung fields should be carried out regularly in patients with ACS to assess for evidence of heart failure. Clinical manifestations of acute heart failure include:

- breathlessness
- third heart sound
- sinus tachycardia
- pulmonary rales – at first basal but potentially extending throughout the lung fields
- in some cases, pronounced pulmonary congestion without auscultatory signs (Van de Werf et al 2003).

The Killip classification is widely used and allows the clinician to categorise the degree of heart failure according to clinical findings:

- Class 1 – no rales or third heart sound
- Class 2 – rales over less than 50% of the lung fields, or third heart sound
- Class 3 – rales over 50% of the lung fields
- Class 4 – shock.

In patients with signs of overt heart failure in the acute setting, the following steps should be considered:

- oxygen administration at high concentration (pulse oximetry is recommended)
- morphine or diamorphine intravenously if the patient is distressed
- correction of any rhythm disturbance causing haemodynamic upset
- diuretics

- nitrates (oral or intravenous) titrated according to blood pressure
- early commencement of angiotensin converting enzyme (ACE) inhibitors, unless contraindicated
- inotropic support, haemodynamic monitoring and assisted ventilation, which may be required in severe cases
- whether reperfusion by thrombolysis or PCI is indicated – seek advice from a senior clinician.

The American College of Cardiology/American Heart Association recommend that PCI should be performed in MI patients with severe congestive heart failure and/or pulmonary oedema (Killip class 3 – see above) within 12 h of onset of symptoms (Antman et al 2004). The aim should be a 'medical contact to balloon time' of within 90 min. This situation requires an urgent opinion from a senior clinician.

Cardiogenic shock

Cardiogenic shock represents a failure of the heart adequately to pump oxygenated blood to the tissues. Conditions that predispose patients to cardiogenic shock are listed in Box 6.1. In patients with MI within the last 24 h, the clinical picture may include:

- severe hypotension (systolic BP <90 mmHg)
- low urine output
- signs of poor tissue perfusion (signs might include: cold sweaty skin, cyanosis, and irritability and restlessness due to poor cerebral perfusion)
- tachycardia
- pulmonary oedema.

BOX: **6.1** 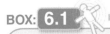 ||||||||||||||||||||||||||||||||||||||||||||||||||||||||||||||||||||||||||

> ### Predisposing conditions for cardiogenic shock
> *(Jowett & Thompson 2004)*
>
> #### Recent massive myocardial infarction
> A lesion in the left main stem coronary artery is the usual culprit resulting in 40–50% of the left ventricular myocardium being damaged.
>
> #### Acute on chronic infarction
> A smaller infarct subsequent to previous infarcts may take the cumulative left ventricular myocardial damage to more than 40%.
>
> #### Myocardial infarction with mechanical complication
> For example, ruptured ventricular septum, ruptured mitral valve or left ventricular aneurysm.
>
> #### Myocardial infarction with recurrent (usually ventricular) arrhythmia
>
> #### Extensive right ventricular infarction (see p. 70)

Emergency PCI or surgery may be life-saving and should be considered at an early stage (Van de Werf et al 2003).

The prognosis of patients with cardiogenic shock is very poor – the best approach is prevention (Jowett & Thompson 2004). Early reperfusion strategies – whether by thrombolysis or primary PCI – help to reduce the risk in MI patients. For those patients who present in cardiogenic shock, emergency PCI is the preferred therapy, or, for patients with severe disease affecting three vessels or the left main stem coronary artery, immediate coronary artery bypass grafts (Hochman 2003).

Treatment

Whilst a detailed discussion of the management of cardiogenic shock in MI is beyond the scope of this book, the key therapeutic features include:

- oxygen at high concentration
- haemodynamic support with inotropic drugs (dopamine and dobutamine), fluids and/or vasodilators, as appropriate
- control of arrhythmias
- early decision regarding suitability for primary PCI or cardiac surgery
- consideration of pulmonary artery catheter, ventilatory support, intra-aortic balloon pump support, left ventricular assist device.

Right ventricular infarction (RVI)

Though RVI can be tolerated well, in the context of inferior STEMI, it may be suspected where the patient develops hypotension with a raised jugular venous pressure and clear lung fields. ST elevation in lead V4R (see Chapter 5) is further evidence of RVI (Haji and Movahed 2000), as are Q waves and ST elevation in leads V1–V3 (Van de Werf et al 2003).

It is important to establish RVI as the cause of hypotension and related clinical signs accurately – management differs from that of shock due to left ventricular impairment. Vasodilators (e.g. diuretics and nitrates), in particular, can make things worse.

Consider:

- rapid IV fluid loading with careful haemodynamic monitoring

- reperfusion: thrombolysis or PCI
- rhythm management.

Ventricular septal defect/rupture

Rupture of the ventricular septal wall occurs in a small number of patients following MI. The clinical presentation is that of heart failure associated with a new pansystolic murmur. The diagnosis can be confirmed through echocardiography and right heart catheterisation. Such patients would normally require urgent surgery, but mortality is high. Supportive therapy may include nitrates, diuretics, inotropes and an intra-aortic balloon pump.

Rupture of the free wall of the left ventricle usually results in circulatory collapse with pulseless electrical activity (PEA). The prognosis is grim.

 References

Antman EM, Anbe DT, Armstrong PW et al 2004 ACC/AHA guidelines for the management of patients with ST-elevation myocardial infarction; A report of the American College of Cardiology/American Heart Association Task Force on Practice Guidelines (Committee to revise the 1999 guidelines for the management of patients with acute myocardial infarction). Journal of the American College of Cardiology 44:E1–E211

Das R, Dorsch M, Lawrance R et al 2005 External validation, extension and recalibration of Braunwald's simple risk index in a community based cohort of patients with both STEMI and NSTEMI. International Journal of Cardiology [E pub ahead of print, May 27].

Haji SA, Movahed A 2000 Right ventricular infarction – diagnosis and treatment. Clinical Cardiology 23:473–482

Hochman JS 2003 Cardiogenic shock complicating acute myocardial infarction: expanding the paradigm. Circulation 107:2998

Jowett NI, Thompson DR 2003 Comprehensive coronary care, 3rd edn. Baillière Tindall, London, p 214

Van de Werf F, Ardissino D, Betriu A et al 2003 The Task Force on the
Management of Acute Myocardial Infarction of the European Society
of Cardiology: management of acute myocardial infarction in patients
presenting with ST-segment elevation. European Heart Journal
24:28–66

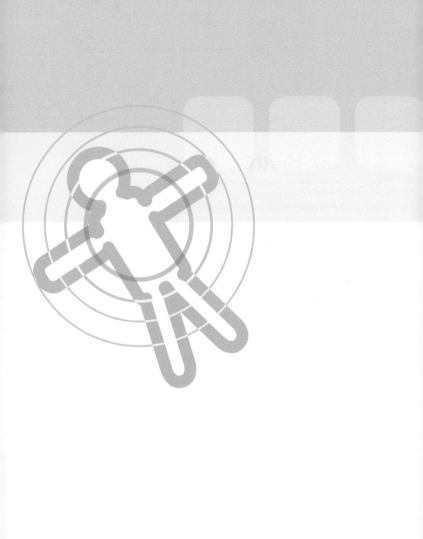

Chapter 7

Cardiac rhythm disturbances and ACS

Chapter contents

Introduction   76

Narrow complex tachycardia   77

Bradycardia   78

First degree heart block   81

Second and third degree AV block   82

Ventricular arrhythmias not normally associated with
cardiac arrest   84

Arrhythmias associated with cardiac arrest   85

This chapter:
- illustrates common arrhythmias that can occur in association with ACS
- outlines management options.

Introduction

Monitoring of the ECG plays a crucial role in the management of the patient with suspected ACS. Changes in cardiac rhythm can happen without warning and can sometimes prove fatal. ECG monitoring should, therefore, be commenced as soon as possible in order to detect life-threatening arrhythmias. The presence of a defibrillator is mandatory in the setting of emergency cardiac care.

Cardiac arrhythmias commonly form part of the clinical picture of patients with ACS – the development of cardiac care units was based on this premise. Patients receiving prompt thrombolysis or PCI seem less likely to develop late-onset or 'secondary' ventricular fibrillation (VF) following STEMI.

An understanding of the normal cardiac cycle and complexities of ECG interpretation are outside the remit of this book, but there are many excellent texts available.

The immediate management of the arrhythmia will be determined by the presence or absence of adverse signs:

- systolic BP < 90 mmHg
- heart rate < 40 beats per minute
- ventricular arrhythmias compromising BP
- heart failure.

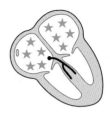

Lead II:

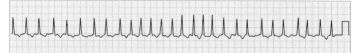

Figure 7.1 ECG of atrial fibrillation. Reproduced with permission from Hampton (2003a).

Narrow complex tachycardia

Tachycardia refers to a heart rate in excess of 100 beats per minute. In *sinus tachycardia* the conduction is essentially normal. The heart rate may be increased because of exercise, emotion or pain, or because of medication or diet (e.g. caffeine) – relatively benign scenarios and easily correctable. Tachycardia associated with adverse signs, however, may indicate a need to identify and correct any underlying cause (e.g. haemorrhage, heart failure, shock or thyroid dysfunction).

Narrow complex tachycardias can include *atrial fibrillation* (if the ventricular response is more than 100 per minute) (Fig. 7.1) and other *supraventricular arrhythmias* (Fig. 7.2). These are not discussed in detail here. Management is dictated largely by the presence of adverse signs (see the algorithm in Fig. 7.3).

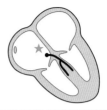

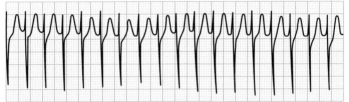

Figure 7.2 ECG of a regular narrow complex tachycardia.
Reproduced with permission from Hampton (2003a).

Bradycardia

Bradycardia refers to a slow heart rate (i.e. less than 60 beats per minute). This may be a normal phenomenon, particularly in the young, fit individual, or may be associated with medication (e.g. beta-blockade). It is also commonly seen in inferior STEMI patients, however, and in those with conduction disorders (heart blocks) and in pre-terminal states.

The presence of adverse signs are an indication for atropine. Consider temporary pacing in resistant cases. See Figure 7.4 for management. Reperfusion is a priority in STEMI patients with atropine-resistant bradycardia.

Sinus bradycardia is a sinus rhythm slower than 60 per minute (Fig. 7.5).

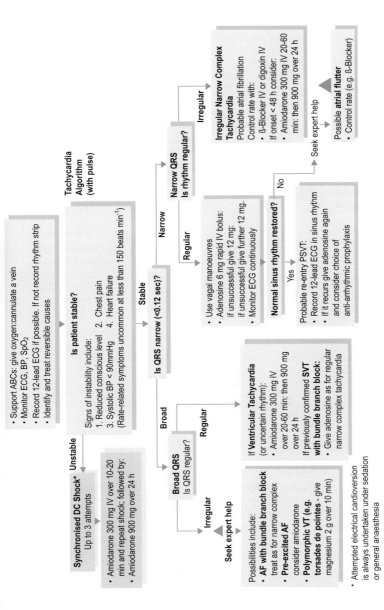

Figure 7.3 Algorithm for tachycardia. Reproduced by permission of Nolan et al (2005).

Tachycardia Algorithm (with pulse)

- Support ABCs: give oxygen;cannulate a vein
- Monitor ECG, BP, SpO₂
- Record 12-lead ECG if possible. If not record rhythm strip
- Identify and treat reversible causes

Is patient stable?

Signs of instability include:
1. Reduced conscious level
2. Chest pain
3. Systolic BP < 90mmHg
4. Heart failure
(Rate-related symptoms uncommon at less than 150 beats min⁻¹)

Unstable

Synchronised DC Shock*
Up to 3 attempts

- Amiodarone 300 mg IV over 10-20 min and repeat shock; followed by:
- Amiodarone 900 mg over 24 h

Stable

Is QRS narrow (<0.12 sec)?

Broad → **Broad QRS** Is QRS regular?

- **Irregular** → Seek expert help

  Possibilities include:
  - **AF with bundle branch block** treat as for narrow complex
  - **Pre-excited AF** consider amiodarone
  - **Polymorphic VT (e.g. torsades de pointes** - give magnesium 2 g over 10 min)

- **Regular** →

  If **Ventricular Tachycardia** (or uncertain rhythm):
  - Amiodarone 300 mg IV over 20-60 min: then 900 mg over 24 h
  If previously confirmed **SVT with bundle branch block:**
  - Give adenosine as for regular narrow complex tachycardia

Narrow → **Narrow QRS** Is rhythm regular?

- **Regular** →

  - Use vagal manoeuvres
  - Adenosine 6 mg rapid IV bolus: if unsuccessful give 12 mg: if unsuccessful give further 12 mg.
  - Monitor ECG continuously

  Normal sinus rhythm restored?

  - **Yes** → Probable re-entry PSVT:
    - Record 12-lead ECG in sinus rhythm
    - If it recurs give adenosine again and consider choice of anti-arrhythmic prophylaxis

  - **No** → Seek expert help
    Possible atrial flutter
    - Control rate (e.g. β-Blocker)

- **Irregular** →

  Irregular Narrow Complex Tachycardia
  Probable atrial fibrillation
  Control rate with:
  - β-Blocker IV or digoxin IV
  If onset < 48 h consider:
  - Amiodarone 300 mg IV 20-60 min: then 900 mg over 24 h
  Seek expert help

* Attempted electrical cardioversion is always undertaken under sedation or general anaesthesia

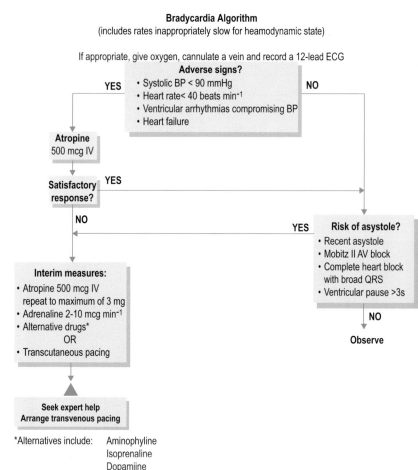

Bradycardia Algorithm
(includes rates inappropriately slow for heamodynamic state)

If appropriate, give oxygen, cannulate a vein and record a 12-lead ECG

Adverse signs?
YES   NO
• Systolic BP < 90 mmHg
• Heart rate< 40 beats min⁻¹
• Ventricular arrhythmias compromising BP
• Heart failure

Atropine
500 mcg IV

Satisfactory   YES
response?

NO

YES   **Risk of asystole?**
• Recent asystole
• Mobitz II AV block
• Complete heart block
  with broad QRS
• Ventricular pause >3s

Interim measures:
• Atropine 500 mcg IV
  repeat to maximum of 3 mg
• Adrenaline 2-10 mcg min⁻¹
• Alternative drugs*
      OR
• Transcutaneous pacing

NO

Observe

Seek expert help
Arrange transvenous pacing

*Alternatives include: Aminophyline
                         Isoprenaline
                         Dopamiine
                         Glucagon (if beta-blocker or calcium-channel blocker overdose)
                         Glycopyrrolate can be used instead of atropine

Figure 7.4 Algorithm for bradycardia. Reproduced by permission of Nolan et al (2005).

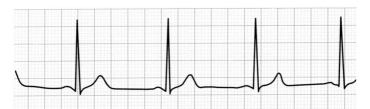

Figure 7.5 ECG of sinus bradycardia. Reproduced with permission from Hampton (2003).

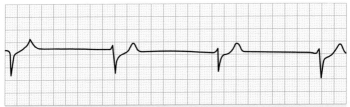

Figure 7.6 ECG of junctional bradycardia. Reproduced with permission from Hampton (2003b).

In *junctional bradycardia*, the impulse originates from the atrioventricular (AV) node or junction and the P wave may be absent, inverted or 'buried' within the QRS complex, or the P–R interval may be shortened (Fig. 7.6). Classically, the associated P wave is upright in lead aVR and negative in lead II.

First degree heart block

This is a benign phenomenon characterised by a prolonged P–R interval (Fig. 7.7) and rarely requires treatment.

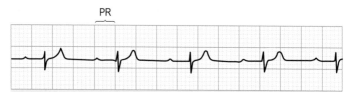

Figure 7.7 ECG of first degree heart block. Reproduced with permission from Hampton (2003a).

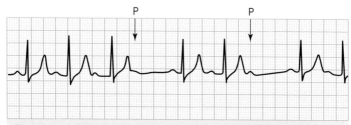

Figure 7.8 ECG of second degree heart block type I (Mobitz 1 or Wenckebach). Reproduced with permission from Hampton (2003b).

Second and third degree AV block

In second degree type 1 AV block (also called Mobitz 1 or Wenkebach), the P–R interval lengthens between beats until a beat is 'dropped'; a cycle that repeats itself, usually without haemodynamic compromise (Fig. 7.8).

In second degree type 2 AV block (Mobitz II), there is more than one P wave for every QRS complex (2:1, 3:1, etc.) but, unlike in type 1, the P–R interval is constant (Fig. 7.9). Adverse signs are more common and there is the risk of deterioration to ventricular standstill in some patients.

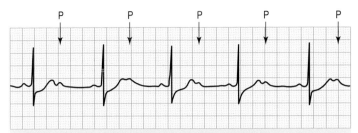

Figure 7.9 ECG of second degree heart block type II (with 2:1 AV block). The hidden P waves are highlighted. Reproduced with permission from Hampton (2003a).

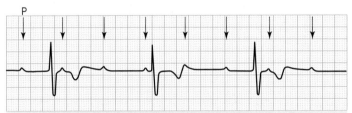

Figure 7.10 ECG of third degree heart block. Reproduced with permission from Hampton (2003a).

In third degree or 'complete' heart block, there is no relationship (association) between atrial and ventricular activity: P waves appear regularly, as do QRS complexes (which tend to be wide and bizarre), but they are independent of one another (Fig. 7.10). This can be well tolerated in the chronic form (especially in older people and those with some congenital heart problems), but can be very serious in the context of an acute event.

In inferior STEMI, asymptomatic second and third degree block tends to resolve in hours or days. In anterior STEMI, second or third degree heart block is associated with a poor outlook.

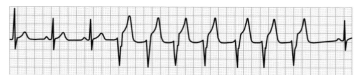

Figure 7.11 Idioventricular rhythm. Reproduced with permission from Hampton (2003a).

ALS guidelines (Nolan et al 2005) recommend that, if adverse signs are present, the patient should be given atropine 500 µg IV (see Fig. 7.4). If the response is unsatisfactory, interim measures should be instigated, such as repeat atropine to a maximum of 3 µg, an adrenaline (epinephrine) infusion or transcutaneous (noninvasive) pacing. Expert help should be sought and transvenous pacing arranged. Even in the absence of adverse signs, Mobitz II and third degree heart block should be treated with interim measures whilst expert help is sought. A key priority in these circumstances is to re-open the occluded coronary artery.

Ventricular arrhythmias not normally associated with cardiac arrest

Idioventricular rhythm

Characterised by wide QRS complexes (> 3 small squares) and a heart rate less than 100 beats per minute, idioventricular rhythm is commonly associated with restoration of blood flow through a coronary artery following thrombolysis (and occasionally following spontaneous reperfusion) (Fig. 7.11). No specific treatment is required in the absence of adverse signs. The rhythm should not be confused with the more malignant ventricular tachycardia (VT).

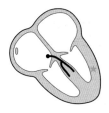

Note

¥ After two sinus beats, the rate increases to 150/min. The QRS complexes become broad, and the T waves are difficult to identify. The final beat shows a return to sinus rhythm

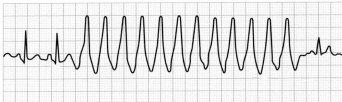

Figure 7.12 Ventricular tachycardia. Reproduced with permission from Jowett & Thompson (1989).

Arrhythmias associated with cardiac arrest

Witnessed ventricular fibrillation (VF) and pulseless VT require immediate DC shocks.

Arrhythmias associated with cardiac arrest can be divided into two groups: shockable rhythms (VF/VT[1]) that require defibrillation, and non-shockable rhythms (asystole and PEA) (Nolan et al 2005).

Shockable rhythms

Ventricular tachycardia (VT)[1]

[1]Note that, whilst VF and pulseless VT *always* require defibrillation, the management of VT *with a pulse* will depend on the patient's ability to tolerate the VT. See Figure 7.3.

Table 7.1 Pharmacological properties and treatment considerations of common drugs used in cardiac arrest and cardiac arrhythmia

Drug	Actions/uses	Dosage/route
*Adrenaline (epinephrine)	Potent alpha and beta-receptor agonist causing vasoconstriction and increased heart rate/contractility	**Cardiac arrest:** 1mg IV every 3–5 min **Peri-arrest:** For resistant bradycardia (if atropine given but no response) ** 2-10 µg min^{-1} ** Also for consideration following atropine, if there is bradycardia with risk of asystole
*Atropine	Blocks parasympathetic activity	**Cardiac arrest:** Asystole or 'slow' PEA (rate <60 min^{-1}): 3 mg IV

Cautions (*irrelevant if cardiac arrest)	Contraindications	Side effects	Comments
Heart disease, diabetes mellitus, hyperthyroidism, hypertension, cerebrovascular disease, angle-closure glaucoma	N/A	Anxiety, tremor, tachycardia, headache, cold extremities	First-line drug in cardiac arrest
Children, elderly and Down syndrome, gastro-	Angle-closure glaucoma, myasthenia gravis	Constipation, bradycardia, followed by tachycardia,	

• continued on next page

Table 7.1 Pharmacological properties and treatment considerations of common drugs used in cardiac arrest and cardiac arrhythmia

Drug	Actions/uses	Dosage/route
Atropine (*cont'd*)	In bradycardia increases sinoatrial and atrioventricular node activity	**Peri-arrest:** For bradycardia with adverse signs and/or risk of asystole: 500 µg IV repeated, if necessary, every 3–5 min (max 3 mg)
*Amiodarone	Works on all phases of the action potential Used in refractory VF or pulseless VT	**VF/VT arrest:** If VF/VT persist after 3 shocks, give 300 mg by bolus injection. Further dose of 150 mg may be given for recurrent or

Cautions (*irrelevant if cardiac arrest)	Contraindications	Side effects	Comments
oesophageal reflux, diarrhoea, ulcerative colitis, myocardial infarction, hypertension, conditions characterised by tachycardia, pyrexia, pregnancy and breast feeding		palpitations and arrhythmias, reduced bronchial secretions, urinary retention and urgency, dilatation of pupils, photophobia, dry mouth, flushing and confusion	
Liver and thyroid function tests before use and every 6 months. Chest X-ray	Sinus bradycardia, sinoatrial block, iodine sensitivity. Avoid intravenous use in severe respiratory failure,	Due to high tissue affinity has numerous side effects including:	In cardiac arrest/ cardiac emergencies pre-filled syringes

• continued on next page

Table 7.1 Pharmacological properties and treatment considerations of common drugs used in cardiac arrest and cardiac arrhythmia

Drug	Actions/uses	Dosage/route
Amiodarone (*cont'd*)	Also used in sustained VT, narrow complex tachycardias, e.g. SVT, atrial fibrillation/flutter	refractory VF/VT, followed by an infusion of 900 mg over 24 h **Tachycardia (with pulse) patient unstable:** Following synchronised DC shocks (up to 3 attempts) 300 mg IV over 10–20 min and repeat shock; followed by 900 mg over 24 h **Patient stable with VT (or uncertain rhythm):** 300 mg IV

Cautions (*irrelevant if cardiac arrest)	Contraindications	Side effects	Comments
before use in heart failure, renal impairment, elderly, severe bradycardia, and in conduction disturbances	severe arterial hypotension	bradycardia and conduction disturbances, hypothyroidism, hyperthyroidism, diffuse pulmonary alveolitis, pneumonitis and fibrosis, jaundice, hepatitis, cirrohosis	are available Incompatible with saline, must be flushed or infused using 5% dextrose Very long half life exceeding several weeks Can prolong Q–T interval

• continued on next page

Table 7.1 Pharmacological properties and treatment considerations of common drugs used in cardiac arrest and cardiac arrhythmia

Drug	Actions/uses	Dosage/route
Amiodarone (*cont'd*)		over 20–60 min; then 900 mg over 24 h (Non-cardiac arrest dosing regimes tend to vary – follow local guidelines)
Adenosine	Blocks adenosine triphosphate (ATP) pump Used to terminate re-entrant tachycardia or diagnosis of broad complex tachycardias	**Peri-arrest:** for narrow complex regular tachycardias in stable patients: 6 mg rapid IV bolus; if unsuccessful give further 12 mg. Monitor ECG continuously. If unsuccessful a further 12 mg can be given

Cautions (*irrelevant if cardiac arrest)	Contraindications	Side effects	Comments
Atrial fibrillation/ flutter with accessory pathways (such as Wolff-Parkinson -White syndrome), heart transplant.	Second or third degree AV block and sick sinus syndrome	Facial flushing, chest pain, dyspnoea, choking sensation, broncho- spasm, severe bradycardia, nausea and	Patients need to be warned of side effects as these can be very distressing

Extremely short duration |

• continued on next page

Table 7.1 Pharmacological properties and treatment considerations of common drugs used in cardiac arrest and cardiac arrhythmia

Drug	Actions/uses	Dosage/route (*irrelevant if cardiac arrest)
Adenosine (cont'd)		(*Dosing regimes tend to vary – follow local guidelines*)

Sources: Nolan JP, Deakin CD, Soar J et al 2005 and BNF 49 (2005). Whilst every effort has been made to ensure the accuracy of information supplied, readers should consult an approved formulary, such as the British National Formulary (BNF), which is updated twice yearly, and can access the latest guidelines at www.bnf.org/

VT has three main characteristics:

- the rate is usually >120 bpm
- it is regular
- QRS complexes are broad (>120 ms) (Fig. 7.12).

Any broad complex (>3 small squares) tachycardia should be considered as ventricular in origin until proven otherwise, following a senior specialist opinion.

Pulseless VT requires immediate defibrillation. See the ALS algorithm on the inside front cover.

VT may not always cause cardiac arrest; short bursts ('salvos') of VT are common in the acute phase of ACS (especially STEMI).

Cautions	Contraindications	Side effects	Comments
		light-headedness	(8–10 s). Needs to be given with rapid flush/infusion

Treatment with drugs such as amiodarone, direct current (DC) cardioversion or 'overdrive' pacing is usually indicated when the VT is sustained. See Figure 7.3 for management and Table 7.1 (see pages 86–95) for drug dosages. Low serum potassium may predispose the patient to ventricular arrhythmias (Sayer et al 2000) and in the setting of STEMI the aim is generally to keep the K^+ above 4.0 mmol/L.

Ventricular fibrillation (VF)

In VF, the rhythm is completely chaotic and there are no discernible complexes to be seen (Fig. 7.13). This rhythm *always* results in cardiac arrest. Immediate defibrillation is mandatory. See the ALS algorithm on the inside front cover.

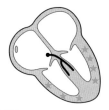

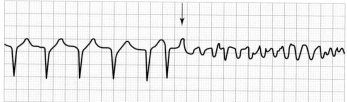

Figure 7.13 Ventricular fibrillation. Reproduced with permission from Hampton (2003a).

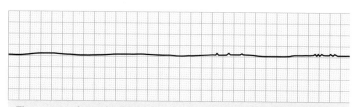

Figure 7.14 Asystole. Reproduced with permission from Jevon (2002).

Non-shockable rhythms

Asystole

Asystole is a complete absence of electrical ventricular activity (Fig. 7.14), though occasionally P waves may be visible (Fig. 7.15). The presence of P waves is an indication for external pacing. See the ALS algorithm on the inside front cover for the

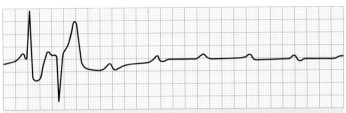
Figure 7.15 P wave asystole. Reproduced with permission from Hampton (2003b).

overall management of asystolic cardiac arrest and Table 7.1 for drug dosages.

Pulseless electrical activity (PEA)

PEA results from the absence of the mechanical pumping action of the heart. Cardiac arrest caused by PEA, therefore, occurs where the monitor displays *any organised electrical activity* that should *normally* produce a pulse but where no pulse is present. A heart rate of less than 60 beats per minute is referred to as 'slow PEA'. Atropine should be given in this scenario. See the ALS algorithm on the inside front cover for overall management of PEA cardiac arrest.

References

Hampton JR 2003a The ECG made easy, 6th edn. Churchill Livingstone, Edinburgh

Hampton JR 2003b The ECG in parctice, 4th edn. Churchill Livingstone, Edinburgh

Jevon P 2002 Advanced cardiac life support: a practical guide. Butterworth-Heinemann, UK

Jowett NI, Thompson DR 1989 Comprehensive coronary care. Baillière Tindall, UK

Nolan JP, Deakin CD, Soar J et al 2005 European Resuscitation Council guidelines for resuscitation 2005, Section 4. Adult advanced life support. Resuscitation 6751:S39–S86

Sayer JW, Archbold RA, Wilkinson P et al 2000 Prognostic implications of ventricular fibrillation in acute myocardial infarction: strategies required for further mortality reduction. Heart 84:258–261

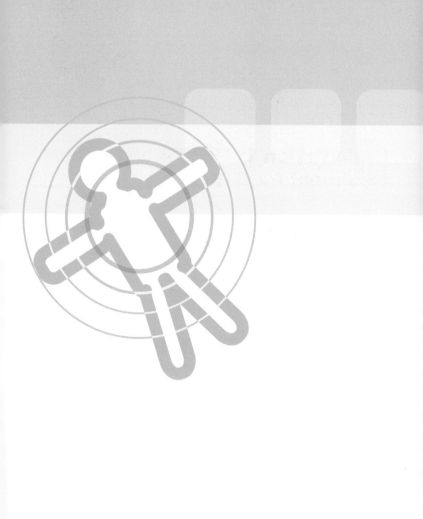

Chapter 8

Reperfusion 1: Thrombolytic treatment for STEMI

Chapter contents

Introduction   102

Thrombolytic drugs   102

Communication   103

Adjunctive therapy: aspirin and heparin   111

This chapter:

- sets out the evidence base and standards for early treatment of STEMI

- highlights key practical issues concerning the use of thrombolytic therapy

- discusses the use of adjunctive therapy.

Introduction

The use of thrombolytic (fibrinolytic) treatment in patients with STEMI has been proven to reduce mortality. The treatment is time dependent – in patients presenting within 3 h of symptom onset, every minute of delay equates with 11 days of life lost (Rawles 1997). Treatment is effective up to 6 h after onset and this may be extended to up to 12 h depending on the presenting features; however, the sooner treatment starts the better. Primary PCI may be the preferred strategy if immediately available and there is evidence of its superiority over thrombolysis in patients presenting more than 3 h from symptom onset (Silber et al 2005). There are national and international standards for rapid treatment. Those set out in the National Service Framework for Coronary Heart Disease (Department of Health 2000), as discussed in Chapter 1, are typical. PCI is discussed in Chapter 9.

Thrombolytic drugs

Four thrombolytic drugs are in common UK usage: streptokinase, alteplase, tenecteplase and reteplase. The ease of use of the latter two agents, which are available for bolus administration, has meant that ambulance crews are increasingly providing this time-dependent treatment before patients reach hospital. In future, it is expected that most thrombolytic treatment will be given before hospital admission, where PCI is not readily available. The key differences between the four available agents are shown in Table 8.1.

The main hazard associated with thrombolytic therapy is bleeding, the most feared complication being intracranial haemorrhage (ICH). This risk increases with age (Gurwitz et al 1998) and lower body weight; higher rates of ICH have been associated with newer agents (Armstrong et al 2001). This risk has to be offset against the substantially higher mortality risk following MI in older patients who do not get reperfusion treatment. Primary PCI is strongly indicated where a patient has a high bleeding risk thrombolysis (Antman et al 2004).

Local policies may differ slightly, but all are designed to 'select out' patients at high risk of haemorrhage (who should then be referred urgently for PCI, as above). Box 8.1 lists the contraindications identified by the European Society of Cardiology (Van de Werf et al 2003). Many centres and cardiac networks have developed checklists to facilitate decision making.

The initial assessment of patients with suspected ACS, the process for rapid identification of those eligible for treatment, and the care of patients receiving thrombolysis are covered elsewhere in this book (Chapters 2, 5 and 9).

Communication

While perhaps incapable of giving informed consent in the circumstances (severe pain and distress, opiate

Table 8.1 Characteristics and administration information of the four thrombolytic drugs licensed for use in the UK in 2005

Thrombolytic drug	Fibrin selective	Price*
Streptokinase (Streptase)	No	£81.18–£89.72
Tenecteplase (TNK) (Metalyse)	Yes	£665 (40 mg/8000 u) £735 (50 mg/10 000 u)

Dosage/drug administration	Half life	Comments
1.5 million units. Given as infusion over 1 h. *Preparation:* Powder vial reconstituted with 10 ml water (for injection) added to 50–200 ml normal saline	23 min	Current UK practice is usually to give only once (NICE, October 2002). Adjuvant heparin therapy not normally required. *Adverse reactions:* • Hypotension (usually < 20 min from commencement) • Allergic/anaphylatic reaction
Rapid single bolus injection over 10 s. *Preparation:* Pack contains 1 pre–filled syringe (water for injection), powder vial for reconstitution and transfer device. *Dose according to patient's weight:* • <60 kg–30 mg (6000 u)	20 min	Requires pre-treatment with heparin 4000–5000 u bolus. Followed by unfractionated heparin (800 u/h–1000 u/h) infusion for 48 h (adjusted according to APTT) (Pre-hospital scenario: refer to local guidelines)

• continued on next page

Table 8.1 Characteristics and administration information of the four thrombolytic drugs licensed for use in UK

Thrombolytic drug	Fibrin selective	Price*
Tenecteplase (cont'd)		
Reteplase (Rapilysin)	Yes	£666.61 (2 vial pack)
normal		

Dosage/drug administration	Half life	Comments
• 60 kg to <70 kg –35 mg (7000 u) • 70 kg to <80 kg –40 mg (8000 u) • 80 kg to <90 kg –45 mg (9000 u) • >90 kg–50 mg (10 000 u) (from summary of product characteristics, Boeringher Ingleheim M10/B/SPC/4 (July 2003))		
Given by 2 × 10 u bolus doses given 30 min between boluses. *Preparation:* Pack contains 2 × vials powder, 2 × pre-filled syringes (water for injection) and transfer	13–16 min	Requires pre-treatment with heparin 5000 u bolus, followed by infusion of 1000 u/h (starting after 2nd reteplase bolus) for min 24 h (pref. 48–72 h). Aim to keep APTT at 1.5–2 × (Pre-hospital scenario: refer

• continued on next page

Table 8.1 Characteristics and administration information of the four thrombolytic drugs licensed for use in UK

Thrombolytic drug	Fibrin selective	Price*
Alteplase (Actylise)	Yes	£300 per 50 mg vial

Adapted from Opie & Gersh 2005 and BNF 49 (2005). Whilst every effort has been made to ensure the accuracy of information supplied, readers should consult an approved formulary, such as the British National Formulary (BNF), which is updated twice yearly, and can access the latest guidelines at www.bnf.org/ for specific prescribing information.

*Prices quoted are from the BNF and may be higher than the actual cost negotiated locally.

Dosage/drug administration	Half life	Comments
Given over 90 min using the following regime: 15 mg bolus followed by 50 mg over 30 min, then 35 mg over 1 h (total 100 mg). *Preparation:* Powder vial reconstituted with 50 ml water for injection and made up into dosages described above	<5 min	Requires pre-treatment with heparin 4000–5000 u bolus. Followed by unfractionated heparin (800 u/h– 1000 u/h) infusion for 48 h (adjusted according to APTT). Complicated dosage regime, now largely replaced by the use of one of the single- or double-bolus alternatives

BOX: 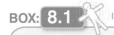 8.1

Contraindications to fibrinolytic therapy

Absolute contraindications
- Haemorrhagic stroke
- Ischaemic stroke or stroke of unknown origin at any time
- Central nervous system damage or neoplasms
- Recent major trauma/surgery/head injury (within preceding 3 weeks)
- Gastrointestinal bleeding within the last month
- Known bleeding disorder
- Aortic dissection

Relative contraindications
- Transient ischaemic attack in preceding 6 months
- Oral anticoagulant therapy
- Pregnancy or within 1 week post partum
- Non-compressible punctures
- Traumatic resuscitation
- Refractory hypertension (systolic blood pressure >180 mmHg)
- Advanced liver disease
- Infective endocarditis
- Active peptic ulcer

Reproduced with permission from: Van de Werf et al 2003

administration, etc.), MI patients should, nevertheless, receive as much information as is reasonable about their care. Many centres use an 'aide-mémoire' to help the clinician provide appropriate information about the benefits and risks of treatment to the patient.

Adjunctive therapy: aspirin and heparin

Aspirin

The importance of the lifesaving role of aspirin in the management of MI has been clearly demonstrated. The ISIS-2 trial (1988) showed that, even when used on its own, aspirin reduces mortality significantly. Soluble aspirin (300 mg) should, therefore, be given (chewed or dissolved in water), irrespective of any previous aspirin taken. Aspirin is very rarely contraindicated in practice. Where patients cannot tolerate aspirin, clopidogrel is the preferred alternative. Clopidogrel has also been reported to be beneficial in *addition* to aspirin in patients with STEMI aged 75 years or less (Sabatine et al 2005), though, at the time of writing, this is not standard practice; refer to local guidelines.

Heparin

The use of unfractionated heparin with thrombolytics (other than streptokinase) has been common practice for many years. The increasing use of low-molecular-weight heparins (LMWH) in the management of NSTEMI ACS has led to consideration of their use as adjuvant treatment for patients receiving thrombolysis for STEMI. Clinical trials of LMWH with thrombolysis have shown a reduction in recurrent ischaemic events, but an increase in major bleeds and ICH, particularly in older patients. Table 8.2 provides a summary of the cautions, contraindications and side-effects of heparin. Always refer to local guidelines.

Table 8.2 Heparin: cautions, contraindications and side-effects

Cautions	Contraindications	Side-effects
Hepatic and renal impairment	Haemophilia and other haemorrhagic disorders	Haemorrhage
Pregnancy		Skin necrosis
Hyperkalaemia	Thrombocytopenia	Thrombocytopenia
Thrombocytopenia	Peptic ulcer	Hyperkaleamia
	Recent cerebral haemorrhage	Hypersensitivity reactions
	Severe hypertension	
	Severe liver disease	
	Major trauma or recent surgery	

Source: Adapted from BNF 49 (2005)

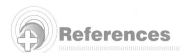 References

Antman E, Anbe DT, Armstrong PW et al 2004 ACC/AHA guidelines for the management of patients with ST-elevation myocardial infarction; a report of the American College of Cardiology/American Heart Association Task Force on Practice Guidelines (Committee to revise the 1999 guidelines for the management of patients with acute myocardial infarction). Journal of the American College of Cardiology 44:E1–E211

Armstrong PW, Granger C, Van de Werf F 2001 Bolus fibrinolysis: risk, benefit, and opportunities. Circulation 103:1171–1173

BNF 2005 British National Formulary 49. British Medical Association & Royal Pharmaceutical Society of Great Britain, London

Department of Health 2000. National service framework for coronary heart disease. Department of Health, London

Gurwitz JH, Gore JM, Goldberg MD et al 1998 Risk for intracranial hemorrhage after tissue plasminogen activator treatment for acute myocardial infarction. Annals of Internal Medicine 129:597–604

ISIS-2 (Second International Study of Infarct Survival) Collaborative Group 1988 Randomised trial of intravenous streptokinase, oral aspirin, both or neither among 17,187 cases of suspected acute myocardial infarction. Lancet 2:349–360

Opie LH, Gersh JB (eds) 2005 Drugs for the heart, 6th edn. Elsevier Saunders, Philadelphia

Rawles JM 1997 Quantification of the benefit of earlier thrombolytic therapy: five-year results of the Grampian Region Early Anistreplase Trial (GREAT). Journal of the American College of Cardiology 30:1181–1186

Sabatine MS, Cannon CP, Gibson CM et al 2005 Addition of clopidogrel to aspirin and fibrinolytic therapy for myocardial infarction with ST segment elevation. New England Journal of Medicine 352:1179–1189

Silber S, Albertsson P, Aviles FF et al 2005 Guidelines for percutaneous coronary interventions: The Task Force for Percutaneous Coronary Interventions of the European Society of Cardiology. European Heart Journal 26:804–847

Van de Werf F, Ardissino D, Betriu A et al 2003 The Task Force on the Management of Acute Myocardial Infarction of the European Society of Cardiology: Management of acute myocardial infarction in patients presenting with ST-segment elevation. European Heart Journal 24:28–66

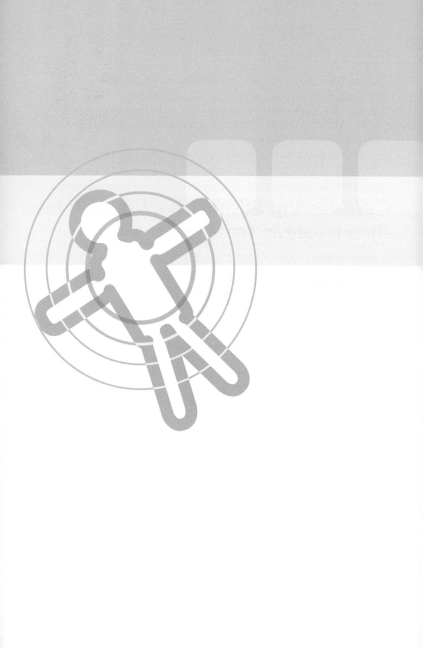

Chapter 9

Care during administration of thrombolytic treatment

Chapter contents

Introduction   116

Beginning treatment   116

Observation   117

Potential complications   118

This chapter:
- provides an overview of care of the STEMI patient receiving thrombolytic treatment.

Introduction

Thrombolytic treatment has been widely available for STEMI for at least two decades; there is, therefore, considerable experience of the clinical course and management of patients receiving this medication.

Thrombolytic treatment reduces mortality and preserves left ventricular function; it does not wholly eliminate the risk of arrhythmia or other complications of MI. Patients may continue to have pain and distress and there may be haemodynamic upset and other adverse events, resulting either from the underlying condition (MI) or the treatment. The key responsibility of the clinician is to observe for signs of change that may require prompt action, while providing the reassurance, dignity, pain relief and information that patients value so much.

The advent of 'third-generation' thrombolytic drugs administered by bolus injection has enabled treatment to begin before STEMI patients reach hospital. Streptokinase use is declining, even in hospital. It can be expected, therefore, that some of the common adverse events associated with streptokinase (allergic reaction, hypotension and bradycardia) will become less common in future. It is also to be expected that most patients in the near future will either have pre-hospital thrombolysis, or primary PCI, if readily available.

Beginning treatment

The initial management of patients with suspected ACS was covered in Chapter 3, and Chapters 2 and 5 considered the selection of patients for thrombolytic treatment. Once the decision has been made to administer a thrombolytic and the relevant local care pathway/protocol has been instituted (whether in or out of hospital, checklists can provide useful aide-mémoires), the drug must be prepared rapidly, and administered in accordance with the product information sheet, remembering the need for adjunctive heparin bolus preceding bolus agents. Baseline observations taken during the initial assessment phase can be compared with subsequent recordings to provide an early warning of deterioration (e.g. sudden drop in BP) or onset of reperfusion (e.g. reduction in ST segment elevation) in response to treatment.

Where adjunctive treatment (discussed in Chapter 8) is required, it is important to emphasise that, where it forms part of the care pathway, heparin treatment should be started promptly. This is particularly relevant to patients who have received thrombolysis before admission to hospital.

Observation

The process of coronary occlusion and reperfusion is dynamic and patients should be observed closely using, where available, continuous ST segment monitoring (or 12-lead ECG recordings, repeated as required), heart rhythm and rate monitoring, blood pressure and respiratory rate measurement. Vital signs monitoring should be very frequent (every 5 min) during the early phase of thrombolytic administration, reducing in frequency as the patient stabilises. Consciousness level should be observed closely for signs of deterioration in the rare event of ICH. Venous puncture sites should be observed for bleeding.

The risk of complications declines over time but most patients should be observed on a cardiac care unit or similar facility for 12–24 h.

Potential complications

The complications of STEMI were discussed in Chapters 6 and 7. The specific adverse events potentially associated with thrombolytic treatment – bleeding, streptokinase-induced hypotension and bradycardia, allergic reactions and recurrent ischaemia or infarction, and reocclusion – are considered below. Rhythm disturbances – mostly benign – may occur in the context of reperfusion and were considered in Chapter 7.

Bleeding

Bleeding is common after thrombolysis and is seen in up to 1 in 10 patients, but is usually restricted to the injection site. Basic measures, such as pressure over puncture sites, should be applied as required. Major bleeding, however, requires discontinuation of the thrombolytic. Antifibrinolytic drugs, such as tranexamic acid and aprotinin, may be required in addition to the administration of coagulation factors (fresh frozen plasma) (BNF 2005). In severe haemorrhage, blood should also be taken for cross matching.

ICH is the most feared complication of thrombolysis. As discussed elsewhere (see Chapter 8, p. 103), the risk is higher in older patients and those with low body weight. The ASSENT 3 Plus Trial (Welsh et al 2005) showed that the overall incidence of ICH associated with pre-hospital thrombolysis was lower when a non-physician initiated the treatment. Scrupulous attention to the patient's blood pressure reduces risk, although rapid reduction using nifedipine 'bites' may be hazardous

(Grossman et al 1996). Adjunctive treatments, such as LMWH, glycoprotein IIb/IIIa inhibitors and clopidogrel all increase risk in the over 75s. ICH as a complication of thrombolysis rarely occurs immediately after administration: in an analysis of the GUSTO-I trial, in those small number of patients who suffered ICH, average (median) time from treatment to ICH was 14 h (Gebel et al 1998).

Hypotension

As streptokinase use declines in UK hospitals, the incidence of a patient developing precipitous hypotension and bradycardia soon after the commencement of the infusion is likely to diminish. This scenario is uncommon with the third-generation bolus agents and extremely unlikely in the ambulance setting.

When hypotension does occur during a streptokinase infusion the patient is usually rapidly symptomatic: mentally obtunded, pre-syncopal, pale, cold and clammy and often very bradycardic. Immediate management involves laying the patient flat, stopping the infusion, removing any buccal or patch nitrates, and administering supplementary oxygen if not already done (unusual in the case of a patient with acute STEMI). Atropine should be used to increase the heart rate as necessary, up to a maximum of 3 mg intravenously. Senior advice should be sought urgently regarding early resumption of the infusion or use of an alternative reperfusion strategy (PCI if readily available).

Allergic reaction

Allergic reaction is mostly associated with streptokinase and the measures outlined for hypotension above – especially stopping the infusion – should be instituted as required. Key signs and symptoms include rash, flushing, wheezing, and loin or lower back pain. Patients may require antihistamine (e.g. chlorpheniramine) and steroid (e.g. hydrocortisone) by injection. Adrenaline (epinephrine) may be required in severe cases. Again, the fact that the patient requires urgent reperfusion should not be forgotten and PCI might be an appropriate option.

Recurrent ischaemia, infarction and reocclusion

These three issues are considered together here not because they are complications of thrombolysis *per se* but because optimal care of the STEMI patient who has received thrombolysis includes vigilance regarding the efficacy of treatment. If thrombolysis does *not* result in resolution of ST segments within 90 min then the patient should be assessed, as a matter of urgency, regarding suitability for transfer for 'rescue' PCI. The 12-lead ECG should, therefore, be recorded routinely 60–90 min from the start of thrombolytic administration. Recurrent or ongoing pain, or return of ST segment elevation (unless in the very early minutes following thrombolytic administration when it is probably a sign of reperfusion), are also indications for assessment by a senior clinician and consideration of PCI.

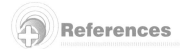 **References**

BNF 2005 British National Formulary 49. British Medical Association & Royal Pharmaceutical Society of Great Britain, London

Gebel JM, Sila CA, Sloan MA et al 1998 Thrombolysis-related intracranial hemorrhage: a radiographic analysis of 244 cases from the GUSTO-I trial with clinical correlation. Global utilization of streptokinase and tissue plasminogen activator for occluded coronary arteries. Stroke 29:563–569

Grossman E, Messerli FH, Grodzicki T et al 1996 Should a moratorium be placed on sublingual nifedipine capsules given for hypertensive emergencies and pseudoemergencies? Journal of the American Medical Association 276:1328–1331

Welsh RC, Chang WC, Goldstein P et al 2005 Time to treatment and the impact of a physician on pre-hospital management of acute ST elevation myocardial infarction:insights from the ASSENT-3 PLUS trial. Heart 91:1400–1406

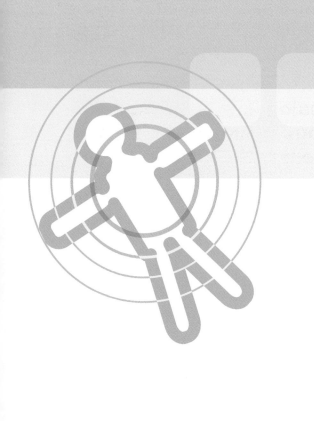

Reperfusion 2: Interventional cardiology in the treatment of the patient with STEMI

Chapter contents

Introduction   124

Potential advantages of primary PCI over thrombolysis therapy in STEMI   124

Primary PCI service models   129

Optimising patency – drug-eluting stents and adjunctive therapy   130

This chapter:

- defines key terms

- briefly describes the growing role of interventional cardiology in the management of patients with ACS, including STEMI

- relates the current 'thrombolysis versus PCI discussion'

- discusses primary PCI service models

- briefly describes adjunctive therapies used in primary PCI.

Introduction

Over recent decades major improvements in both equipment and techniques have enabled many thousands of patients with obstructed or narrowed coronary arteries to benefit from non-surgical treatments, such as angioplasty and stent insertion, known under the umbrella term *percutaneous coronary intervention* (PCI) (Box 10.1). Clear benefits from early (within 48 h of presentation) angiography and PCI have been shown for those ACS patients with high risk features, such as those discussed in Chapter 11.

Potential advantages of primary PCI over thrombolysis therapy in STEMI

The use of PCI techniques in the immediate management of patients with STEMI is growing, following clear evidence that patients have better outcomes with primary PCI compared with hospital thrombolytic treatment (Keeley et al 2003). The

BOX: 10.1 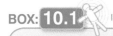 ‖‖

Percutaneous coronary interventions

Angiogram

A procedure in which a fine catheter is inserted via a blood vessel to inject X-ray opaque dye into the coronary arteries to obtain an X-ray image of the anatomy of the coronary arteries.

Angioplasty

A procedure in which a small balloon on the end of a catheter is inserted into an artery (the coronary arteries in CHD) and inflated to widen a narrowed artery (Fig. 10.1 and 10.2).

Stent

An artificial structure inserted into a coronary artery following angioplasty to support the vessel wall and reduce the risk of re-occlusion (Fig. 10.3).

Definitions from Department of Health (2000).

technique and potential effectiveness of balloon angioplasty in reopening coronary arteries are demonstrated in Figures 10.1 and 10.2. Whether the terms 'primary', 'facilitated' or 'rescue PCI' are utilised depends on the timing of the intervention and whether it is preceded by thrombolytic treatment (Box 10.2).

Although the superiority of PCI over very early (within 3 h of onset) thrombolysis in reducing mortality from STEMI is less well determined, PCI is considered by many to be the treatment of first choice if readily available, in part due to the lower risk of ICH and other major cardiac events (Van de Werf et al 2003, Antman et al 2004, Silber et al 2005). One recent NHS assessment of the evidence concluded that, if both thrombolysis and PCI were available routinely, then economic analysis favours PCI, but that, given capacity and staffing constraints in the 'real world' setting, pre-hospital thrombolysis, with transfer

Technique of balloon angioplasty				
Placement of guiding catheter	Introduction of guidewire and crossing of the lesion	Introduction of balloon catheter, with placement across the lesion	Inflation of the balloon catheter	Deflation and removal of the balloon catheter
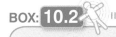				

Figure 10.1 Technique of balloon angioplasty. Reproduced by permission of Crawford, DiMarco & Paulus (2004).

BOX: **10.2**

Percutaneous coronary interventions

Primary PCI
Immediate intervention in the culprit vessel without prior thrombolytic therapy.

Facilitated PCI
A planned intervention undertaken soon after thrombolysis.

Rescue PCI
Intervention in a coronary artery that remains occluded despite thrombolytic therapy.

for rescue PCI where necessary, may be appropriate while clinical networks develop PCI services on an incremental basis (Hartwell et al 2005).

In comparison to (mainly hospital) thrombolysis, primary PCI has been shown to be superior in terms of more effective restoration of coronary blood flow, less recurrent ischaemia, less reocclusion and reinfarction, improved residual left ventricular

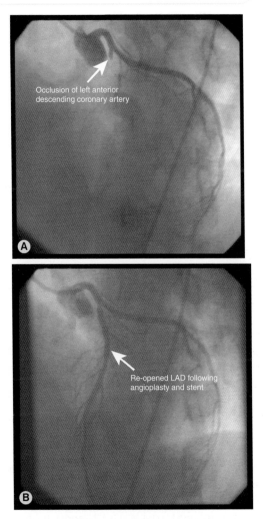

Figure 10.2 Occlusion of left anterior descending
(LAD) coronary artery (A) successfully reopened
following angioplasty and insertion of stent (B).

Delivery of a balloon expandable stent

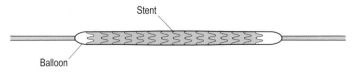

Deflated balloon with premounted stent

Stent

Balloon

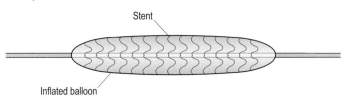

Delivery of stent with inflation of balloon

Stent

Inflated balloon

Figure 10.3 Balloon-delivered stent. Reproduced by permission of Crawford, DiMarco & Paulus (2004).

function and less intracranial haemorrhage. In particular, women and older patients stand to gain from PCI, compared to thrombolysis (Silber et al 2005).

Primary PCI may be of particular benefit where an MI patient is ineligible to receive thrombolysis because of contraindications, such as severe hypertension, advanced age, or late presentation after symptom onset, since outcomes in such cases are much worse than in patients who are eligible to receive thrombolysis (Cohen et al 2003). MI patients who did *not* meet eligibility criteria for a thrombolysis trial had a 12-month mortality twice that of eligible patients (Bjorklund et al 2004). Emergency PCI may be lifesaving in patients with cardiogenic shock (Silber et al 2005).

Both the American Heart Association and the European Society of Cardiology recommend the use of primary PCI, for patients presenting with STEMI, where the delay from first medical contact to balloon is 90 min or less (Antman et al 2004, Van de Werf et al 2003).

In addition to the patient groups discussed above primary PCI is also preferred, if facilities are available, in the following scenarios:

- heart failure (Killip class ≥ 3)
- where diagnosis of STEMI is in doubt (Antman et al 2004).

Primary PCI service models

It is possible that, in the future, a move to wider use of primary PCI for STEMI will result in the development of 'regional heart attack centres' or a that a network of 'STEMI' and 'NSTEMI' hospitals will be established with relevant facilities (Moyer et al 2004).

In the DANAMI 2 trial (Andersen et al 2003), patients in Denmark were assessed following admission to the local district general hospital before being transferred to a PCI centre. In the future, in the UK, ambulance personnel will play a key role in reducing treatment delay by assessing patients for reperfusion, with their decisions based on patient characteristics and locally agreed protocols. It has been suggested that paramedics could safely and effectively expedite access to a PCI centre *without* the need for admission to a non-interventional hospital (Quinn & Whitbread 2005).

Optimising patency – drug-eluting stents and adjunctive therapy

Once the coronary artery is opened, the objective is to maintain patency. Drug-eluting stents are coated with a slow-release drug formulation and have been reported to reduce the risk of restenosis (Kastrati et al 2005). There is ongoing debate about the long-term benefits of such treatments, compared with coronary bypass grafting, in patients with severe coronary disease (Hill et al 2004, Taggart 2005), although the relevance of these findings to patients with STEMI is uncertain.

Drug therapy is crucial in helping to both establish and maintain coronary patency. All patients undergoing PCI should receive aspirin, clopidogrel and heparin (unless contraindicated). Glycoprotein IIb/IIIa inhibitors should be considered in STEMI patients as an adjunctive treatment to PCI (see Chapter 11).

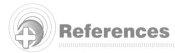

References

Andersen HR, Nielsen TT, Rasmussen K et al (DANAMI-2 Investigators) 2003 A comparison of coronary angioplasty with fibrinolytic therapy in acute myocardial infarction. New England Journal of Medicine 349:733–742

Antman E, Anbe DT, Armstrong PW et al 2004 ACC/AHA guidelines for the management of patients with ST-elevation myocardial infarction; a report of the American College of Cardiology/American Heart Association task force on practice guidelines (Committee to revise the 1999 guidelines for the management of patients with acute myocardial infarction). Journal of the American College of Cardiology 44:E1–E211

Bjorklund E, Lindahl B, Stenestrand U 2004 Outcome of ST-elevation myocardial infarction treated with thrombolysis in the unselected population is vastly different from samples of eligible patients in a large-scale clinical trial. American Heart Journal 148:566–573

Cohen M, Gensini GF, Maritz F et al (TETAMI investigators) 2003 Prospective evaluation of clinical outcomes after acute ST elevation myocardial infarction in patients who are ineligible for reperfusion therapy: preliminary results from the TETAMI registry and randomised trial. Circulation 108 (Suppl. I):III 14–21

Crawford MH, DiMarco JP, Paulus WJ (eds) 2004 Cardiology, 2nd edn. Mosby, Edinburgh

Department of Health 2000 National service framework for coronary heart disease. Department of Health, London

Hartwell D, Colquitt J, Loveman E et al 2005 Clinical effectiveness and cost-effectiveness of immediate angioplasty for acute myocardial infarction: systematic review and economic evaluation. Health Technology Assessment 9:1–99, iii–iv

Hill R, Bagust A, Bakhai A et al 2004 Coronary artery stents: a rapid systematic review and economic evaluation. Health Technology Assessment 8:iii–iv,1–242

Kastrati A, Mehilli J, von Beckerath N et al (ISAR-DESIRE Study Investigators) 2005 Sirolimus-eluting stent or paclitaxel-eluting stent vs balloon angioplasty for prevention of recurrences in patients with coronary in-stent restenosis: a randomized controlled trial. Journal of the American Medical Association 293:165–171

Keeley E, Boura J, Grines C 2003 Primary angioplasty versus intravenous thrombolytic therapy for acute myocardial infarction: a quantitative review of 23 randomised trials. Lancet 361:13–20

Moyer P, Feldman J, Levine J et al 2004 Implications of the mechanical (PCI) vs thrombolytic controversy for ST segment elevation myocardial infarction on the organisation of emergency medical services: the Boston EMS experience. Critical Pathways in Cardiology 3:53–61

Quinn T, Whitbread M 2005 Reduction of treatment delay in patients with ST-elevation myocardial infarction: impact of pre-hospital diagnosis and direct referral to primary percutaneous intervention. European Heart Journal 26:770–777

Silber S, Albertsson P, Aviles F et al 2005 The Task Force for percutaneous coronary interventions of the European Society of Cardiology: guidelines for percutaneous coronary interventions. European Heart Journal 26:804–847

Taggart DP 2005 Surgery is the best intervention for severe coronary artery disease. British Medical Journal 330:785–786

Van de Werf F, Ardissino D, Betriu A et al 2003 The Task Force on the Management of Acute Myocardial Infarction of the European Society of Cardiology: management of acute myocardial infarction in patients presenting with ST-segment elevation. European Heart Journal 24:28–66

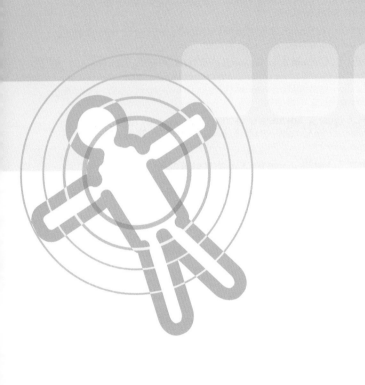

Chapter 11

The non-STEMI patient with ACS

Chapter contents

Introduction   134

Management   135

Other adjunctive treatment: beta blockers and

nitrates   137

This chapter:

- highlights the importance of early risk stratification in ACS

- describes the early management of the patient with non-STEMI ACS

- compares available medicines used in ACS treatment.

Introduction

Non-STEMI (NSTEMI) presentations of ACS account for an estimated 120 000 hospital admissions annually (British Cardiac Society 2001). Twice as many patients are discharged with a diagnosis of 'unstable angina' than have confirmed MI (Fox et al 2000). The condition is certainly not benign: of ACS patients, those with NSTEMI have the highest mortality, with 13% dead at six months (Fox 2004).

As discussed in Chapter 1, the term 'acute coronary syndrome' (ACS) describes a spectrum of conditions sharing a common underlying pathophysiology: obstruction of coronary blood flow due to thrombus following disruption of coronary artery plaque (see Fig.1.2, p 6). The main classifications of ACS relate to changes in the ECG and release of markers of myocardial necrosis: ST segment elevation MI (STEMI), non-ST elevation MI (NSTEMI) and unstable angina (see Fig. 1.3, p 6).

NSTEMI patients at particularly high risk of death or further adverse events (e.g. STEMI) tend to be older (70 years of age and over) and have ST depression or bundle branch block on the admission ECG. Compared to patients under 60 years of age or with normal ECGs, such patients have a three- to fivefold higher risk (Collinson et al 2000). Clinical characteristics of patients at

BOX: 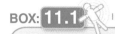 ||||||||||||||||||||||||||||||||||||||||||||||||||||||||||||||||||

The clinical characteristics of patients at high risk of progression to myocardial infarction or death

(Bertrand et al 2002)

- Recurrent ischaemia – either recurrent chest pain or dynamic ST-segment changes (in particular ST segment depression or transient ST-segment elevation)
- Early post-infarction unstable angina
- Elevated troponin levels
- Haemodynamic instability within the observation period
- Major arrhythmias (repetitive ventricular tachycardia, ventricular fibrillation)
- Diabetes mellitus
- An ECG pattern which precludes assessment of ST-segment changes

high risk of dying or progressing to STEMI are summarised in Box 11.1.

A variety of risk-scoring systems have been developed for early identification of patients at high risk of death or other adverse events, facilitating prompt medical treatment or referral for assessment for PCI (see Chapter 10 on PCI). These are summarised in Table 11.1.

Management

Once a diagnosis of STEMI has been excluded on assessment of ECG and clinical features, patients with a history or other features suggestive of ACS require specialised observation in a CCU or equivalent facility. Data from the National Audit of Myocardial Infarction (MINAP) suggest that a minority of

Table 11.1 Summary of predictive variables in identifying 'at-risk' patients presenting with non-ST segment elevation ACS

TIMI risk score for unstable angina/ non-ST elevation MI *(Antman et al 2000)*	GRACE – predictors of hospital mortality *(Granger et al 2003)*
Age >65 years	Killip class
Presence of at least three risk factors for coronary artery disease (family history, hypertension, raised cholesterol, diabetes or active smoker)	Systolic blood
	Heart rate
	Age
	Serum creatinine
Significant coronary stenosis (e.g. prior coronary stenosis >50%)	Cardiac arrest (at presentation)
	ST segment depression
Aspirin use within previous 7 days	Elevated cardiac enzymes
ST depression >0.5mm at presentation	
Severe anginal symptoms (e.g. two or more anginal events in last 24 hours)	
Elevated serum cardiac enzymes	
For further information and a downloadable risk calculator see www.timi.org	For further information and a downloadable risk calculator see www.outcomes-umassmed.org/grace/

NSTEMI patients are admitted to a CCU and that this situation requires a change in practice (Quinn et al 2005). Clinicians should be constantly aware that an initially normal ECG does not wholly rule out MI. Recurrent pain or haemodynamic instability represents an emergency requiring immediate specialist assessment.

General supportive care includes analgesia and oxygen as appropriate. Continuous ST segment monitoring (where available) and ECG rhythm monitoring should be instituted. A defibrillator should be readily available. Following the onset of symptoms, biochemical markers should be measured at appropriate intervals (Table 11.2).

Cardiac markers have been evaluated in the ambulance setting (Svensson et al 2004), but this is not yet in widespread practice in pre-hospital care in the UK. The potential benefit to patients from assessment of marker release very early in the clinical course merits further investigation.

Patients with NSTEMI presentations do not benefit from thrombolytic treatment. Antithrombotic treatment with aspirin, clopidogrel and heparin forms the cornerstone of early management, with glycoprotein IIb/IIIa inhibitors generally reserved for patients identified as at high risk and used in association with an interventional strategy (Table 11.3). A patient pathway depending on risk stratification has been proposed by the European Society of Cardiology (Fig. 11.1) (Silber et al 2005).

Other adjunctive treatment: beta blockers and nitrates

Whilst there is little evidence for the use of either beta blockers or nitrates to reduce mortality in patients with unstable angina,

Table 11.2 Characteristics of commonly used markers of myocardial injury

Marker	Molecular weight (Da)	Range of time to initial elevation (hours)
Myoglobin	17 800	1–4
Troponin I	23 500	6–12
Troponin T	33 000	3–12
Creatinine Kinase (CK)-MB	86 000	3–12
CK-MB tissue isoform	86 000	6–10
Lactate dehydrogenase (LDH)	135 000	10

Reproduced with permission from Crawford, DiMarco & Paulus (2004).

Mean time to peak elevation without recanalisation (hours)	Time to return to normal range	Most common sampling schedule
6	24 h	Admission and every 2 h
24	5–10 days	Admission and 6–9 h
12–48	5–14 days	Admission and 6–9 h
24	48–72 h	Admission and 6–9 h
24	?	Admission and every 2 h
24–48	10–14 days	24 h after onset

Table 11.3 Summary of the pharmacological properties and dosages of antithrombotic therapy

Drug	Action	Loading dose	Maintenance dose
Aspirin	Inhibits thromboxane A_2 receptor	300mg	75 mg
Clopidogrel	Inhibits binding of ADP to platelet receptor	300 mg	75 mg
Gp IIb/IIIa	Inhibit the glycoprotein		
Abciximab	Gp IIb/IIIa platelet receptor	0.25 mg/kg (10–60 min prior to PCI) For unstable angina start up to 24 h before	0.125 μg/kg/min (max. 10 μg/min)
Tirofiban		0.4 μg/kg/min for 30 min	0.1 μg/kg/min

Duration of treatment	Side effects	Notes
Life long	Gastrointestinal disturbances and gastrointestinal bleed (4–5% of patients)	Some of the gastrointestinal effects may be ameliorated by taking with food
9–12 months	Similar to aspirin. Increased risk of extracranial bleeds	In elective CABG, should be stopped 5–7 days prior to surgery
12 h (max. 24 h for unstable angina)	Increased risk of bleed	All are given intravenously. Most benefit is seen in high-risk patients. It is important to check platelet count prior to and after treatment
≥ 48 h (108 h max.)	Thrombocytopenia	For Tirofiban and eptifibatide reduce dose in

• continued on next page

Table 11.3 Summary of the pharmacological properties and dosages of antithrombotic therapy

Drug	Action	Loading dose	Maintenance dose
Eptifibatide		180 µg/kg	2 µg/kg/min
Low-molecular-weight heparin	Binds and catalyses antithrombin-III & thrombin		
Dalteparin	Inhibits clotting factor Xa	120 u/kg every 12 hours (Max. 10000 u 2×/day)	
Enoxaparin*		Start dose same as maintenance dose	1 mg/kg every 12 h

Source: Opie & Gersh (2005). Reproduced with permission. While every effort has been made to ensure the accuracy of information, readers should consult an approved formulary, such as the British National Formulary (BNF) for specific prescribing information.

Duration of treatment	Side effects	Notes
72 h (max.) (96 h max. if PCI during treatment)		patients with reduced creatinine clearance: <30–<50 ml/min
	Heparin-induced haemorrhage	
Up to 8 days. (Check BNF if > 8 days)	Thrombocytopenia	Dalteparin and enoxaparin given by deep **subcutaneous** injection **not intramuscular** injection
Min. 2 days Continued up to 8 days	*Risks for bleeding include severe renal impairment (creatinine clearance <30 ml/min), age, female, use with NSAID, aspirin and clopidogrel	

Table 11.4 Pharmacological properties and treatment considerations for beta blockers and nitrates

Drug	Mode of action	Treatment target	Cautions
Beta blockers *Most commonly used:* Atenolol Metoprolol Bisoprolol[1] Carvedilol[1]	Reduce heart rate by selective inhibition of β1 receptors in myocardium; therefore reduce myocardial oxygen demand. Also inhibit β2 receptors in peripheral vasculature, bronchus, liver and pancreas	Heart rate 50–60bpm In high-risk ACS patients IV route preferred for initial dose[2]	Obstructive airways disease AV block Renal impairment Diabetes History of hypersensitivity
Nitrates	Venodilation producing decrease in myocardial	Treatment is titrated to achieve symptomatic	Severe hepatic or renal impairment Hypothyroidism Hypothermia

Contra-indications	Side effects	Comments
Asthma	Bronchospasm	Dosages depend on type used.
Uncontrolled heart failure	Heart failure	Low-dose, short-acting beta blockers can be used where tolerance may be a problem
Marked bradycardia	Bradycardia	
Sick sinus syndrome	AV block	
Second or third degree AV block	Hypotension	
Hypotension	Peripheral vasoconstriction, exacerbation of intermittent claudication	
Severe peripheral vascular disease		
Known hypersensitivity	Headache	Problems associated with nitrate tolerance can occur. These are related to both the
Hypovolaemia	Flushing	
Hypertrophic	Dizziness	
	Hypotension	

• continued on next page

Table 11.4 Pharmacological properties and treatment considerations for beta blockers and nitrates

Drug	Mode of action	Treatment target	Cautions
Nitrates (*cont'd*)	preload and left ventricular end-diastolic volume leading to a decrease in myocardial oxygen consumption. In addition, nitrates dilate normal and atherosclerotic coronary arteries, increase coronary collateral flow, and inhibit platelet aggregation	relief of chest pain. IV route is preferred during the initial acute stage	Cerebral haemorrhage

[1]*these beta blockers can be used in stable heart failure*
[2]*requires close monitoring of patients and use of cardiac monitor*
Source: Bertrand et al (2002), BNF 49 (2005). Whilst every effort has been made to ensure the accuracy of information, readers should consult an approved formulary, such as the British National Formulary (BNF), for specific prescribing information.

Contra-indications	Side effects	Comments
obstructive cardiomyopathy	Tachycardias (or paradoxical bradycardia)	dosage and duration of treatment. When symptoms are controlled, intravenous nitrates should be replaced with oral nitrates. The timing of prescription should allow for appropriate nitrate-free intervals. Alternative drugs which can be used are potassium-channel activators such as nicorandil
Aortic stenosis		
Cardiac tamponade		
Constrictive pericarditis		
Mitral stenosis		

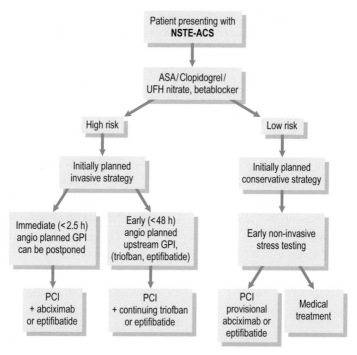

Figure 11.1 Flow chart for planning coronary angiography and PCI. Reproduced with permission from Silber et al (2005).

there is evidence that beta blockers reduce mortality in MI. For this reason, and because of pathophysiological considerations and clinical experience with the use of both drugs in the management of patients with CHD, in the absence of contraindications (see Table 11.4 on pages 144–147) beta blockers and nitrates are recommended for use in patients with NSTEMI ACS (Bertrand et al 2004). In those patients who cannot tolerate beta blockers because of asthma, a non-dihydropyridine calcium channel blocker, such as diltiazem or verapamil, can be used as an alternative.

Identification of those patients presenting with
suspected ACS – particularly those with high risk features
– from the very large numbers presenting with chest pain
presents a challenge to those providing emergency care.
Early triage and treatment by paramedics can help to
minimise delay and ensure effective treatments (e.g. aspirin,
clopidogrel, glycoprotein IIb/IIIa inhibitors) are given
where appropriate at an early stage. The development and
use of clinical pathways supported by evidence-based
guidelines can help clinical teams to manage this complex
group of patients effectively and ensure those at high risk
receive timely access to specialist advice, coronary angiography
and intervention and subsequent secondary prevention and
rehabilitation.

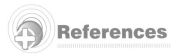

References

Antman EM, Cohen M, Bernink PJ et al 2000 The TIMI risk score for
unstable angina/non-ST elevation MI: a method for prognostication and
therapeutic decision making. Journal of the American Medical Association
284:835–842

Bertrand M, Simoons M, Fox KA et al 2002 The Task Force on the
Management of Acute Coronary Syndromes of the European Society
of Cardiology: management of acute coronary syndromes in patients
presenting without persistent ST-segment elevation. European Heart
Journal 23:1809–1840

British Cardiac Society 2001 Guidelines and Medical Practice Committee,
and Royal College of Physicians Clinical Effectiveness and Evaluation Unit:
Guideline for the management of patients with acute coronary syndromes
without persistent ECG ST segment elevation. Heart 85:133–142

BNF 2005 British National Formulary 49. British Medical Association and
Royal Pharmaceutical Society of Great Britain, London

Collinson J, Flather M, Fox KA et al 2000 Clinical outcomes, risk
stratification and practice patterns of unstable angina and myocardial
infarction without ST elevation: Prospective Registry of Acute Ischaemic
Syndromes in the UK (PRAIS-UK). European Heart Journal
21:1450–1457

Fox KA 2004 Management of acute coronary syndromes: an update. Heart 90:698–706

Fox KA, Cokkinos DV, Deckers J et al 2000 The ENACT study: a pan-European survey of acute coronary syndromes. European Network for Acute Coronary Treatment. European Heart Journal 21:1440–1449

Granger CB, Goldberg RJ, Dabbous O et al (Global Registry of Acute Coronary Events (GRACE) Investigators) 2003 Predictors of hospital mortality in the global registry of acute coronary events. Archives of Internal Medicine 163:2345–2353

Opie LH, Gersh JB (eds) 2005 Drugs for the heart, 6th edn. Elsevier Saunders, Philadelphia

Quinn T, Weston C, Birkhead J et al 2005 The changing role of the coronary care unit: observations from patients admitted to hospitals in England and Wales, 2003–2004. Quarterly Journal of Medicine 98: 797–802

Silber S, Albertsson P, Aviles F et al 2005 The Task Force for Percutaneous Coronary Interventions of the European Society of Cardiology: Guidelines for percutaneous coronary interventions. European Heart Journal 26:804–847

Svensson L, Axelsson C, Nordlander R et al 2004 Prognostic value of biochemical markers, 12-lead ECG and patient characteristics amongst patients calling for an ambulance due to a suspected acute coronary syndrome. Journal of Internal Medicine 255:469–477

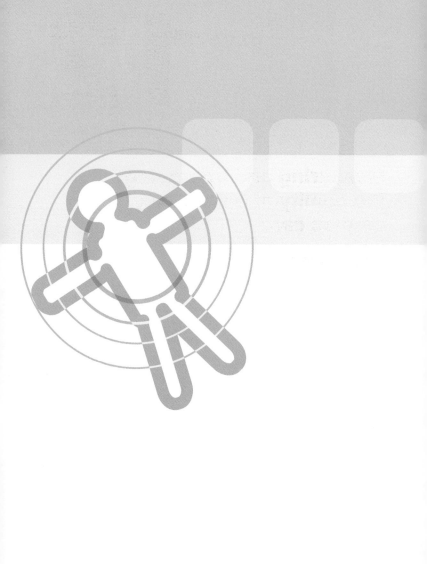

Chapter 12

Measuring and improving the quality of emergency cardiac care

Chapter contents

Introduction   154

Process or outcome?   155

MINAP   155

Using information to improve care   157

This chapter:

- highlights the importance of using robust information to measure and improve the quality of care

- discusses the use of process versus outcome measures to measure quality

- provides an overview of the national audit of myocardial infarction (MINAP) project involving all acute hospitals in England and Wales

- introduces techniques used to support service improvement.

Introduction

As discussed in Chapter 1, governments and professional societies have set a range of national and international standards against which care for patients with ACS can be measured. In the management of STEMI patients, the standards set out in the NSF (Department of Health 2000), as shown in Box 1.1 (p 8), relate to the availability of a defibrillator, the use of aspirin and thrombolytic treatment where indicated and the use of secondary prevention medication. Similar standards have been published by the devolved administrations in Scotland (Scottish Executive 2002) and Wales (National Assembly for Wales 2001).

Standards for PCI in patients with STEMI have been published by the American Heart Association (Antman et al 2004) and the European Society of Cardiology (Van de Werf et al 2003), as discussed in Chapters 1 and 10. Guidelines for the care of patients without persistent ST segment elevation have also been published by these respected authorities.

Having clear, published (and preferably evidence-based) standards and guidelines gives clinicians and managers – and patients – at local level the opportunity to measure their performance and benchmark against similar systems. This measurement and reporting can also be used to identify and remedy any deficiencies in local systems of care. Clinical audit, enabling systematic assessment and improvement in quality of care, is regarded as an essential requirement for all clinicians (Birkhead 2000).

Process or outcome?

Assessing performance using 'hard' outcome data, such as mortality rates, is an imperfect science. While the goals of ACS care are clearly focused on reducing mortality and morbidity, it has been suggested that over 70 years of data collection on patients admitted with AMI would be required to give an accurate reflection of the quality of care (Mant & Hicks 1995). Comparison of hospitals serving similar populations on the basis of AMI mortality rates has largely been abandoned as a means of monitoring standards. Difficulties in the use of hospital mortality data as a performance indicator following cardiac arrest have also been identified (Norris et al 2004). Measures of the process of caring for patients with ACS, rather than the outcomes, are therefore widely used as a surrogate for survival.

MINAP

In England and Wales, the national audit of myocardial infarction project (MINAP) has been established as a response to the NSF. MINAP has built on the experience of earlier multicentre audits (Birkhead 1997, Quinn et al 2003) and uses a technological platform developed by the Central Cardiac

Audit Database group to provide hospitals and ambulance services with both contemporary online analyses of their performance in the care of patients with ACS and comparisons with national aggregate data. All 230 acute hospitals in England and Wales return data electronically on patients with AMI and, increasingly, other ACS presentations. The MINAP dataset, updated several times from the original (Birkhead et al 1999), is now part of the NHS Data Dictionary, and is approved by the English Information Standards Board. MINAP provides one of the most robust registries of ACS care in the world: an annual data validation exercise is mandatory and data completeness averages above 90%. Information from MINAP has been very influential in changing practice in acute cardiac care, as demonstrated by the improvements in door- and call-to-needle times for thrombolysis, and very high rates of secondary prevention medicine use following AMI (Birkhead et al 2004). Data from MINAP have also helped to improve understanding of the challenges associated with monitoring cardiac arrest outcome (Norris et al 2004) and a national audit of cardiac arrest utilising MINAP methodology is being explored (Weston 2004). An important development has been the collaboration between MINAP and the Ambulance Service Association to ensure that ambulance services are now able to access MINAP data on the clinical course and outcome of patients who have come under their care.

Other examples of observational registries and audits being used to improve the quality of ACS care have been reported, including the US-based National Registry of Myocardial Infarction (French 2000), the CRUSADE quality improvement initiative (Hoekstra et al 2005), the Global Registry of Acute Coronary Events (GRACE; Van de Werf et al 2005) and the Swedish Register of Cardiac Intensive Care (Bjorklund et al 2004). The EMMACE study of ACS-related practice in Yorkshire hospitals (Dorsch et al 2001) and the Nottingham Heart Attack

Register (Packham et al 2000) have also provided valuable insights over several years.

The success of MINAP and other projects of this nature depends largely on the quality and timeliness of data input by nurses, ambulance and audit staff across the NHS (Gamon & Carolan 2002).

Using information to improve care

All of the initiatives outlined above have allowed patients to receive better care, possibly by stimulating local clinicians and managers (as well as policy makers at strategic and national levels) to scrutinise their policies and systems of care to identify areas for remedy. Service improvement methods, including process mapping and the use of statistical process control (Duncan et al 2005), which have gained widespread acceptance in the NHS, can make an important contribution to patient care.

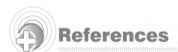

References

Antman E, Anbe DT, Armstrong PW et al 2004 ACC/AHA guidelines for the management of patients with ST-elevation myocardial infarction; a report of the American College of Cardiology/American Heart Association task force on practice guidelines (Committee to revise the 1999 guidelines for the management of patients with acute myocardial infarction). Journal of the American College of Cardiology 44:E1–E211

Birkhead JS 1997 Thrombolytic treatment for myocardial infarction: an examination of practice in 39 United Kingdom hospitals. Myocardial Infarction Audit Group. Heart 78:28–33

Birkhead JS 2000 Responding to the requirements of the national service framework for coronary disease: a core data set for myocardial infarction. Heart 84:116–117

Birkhead JS, Norris RM, Quinn T et al, on behalf of the National Service Framework for Coronary Heart Disease Steering Group 1999 Acute myocardial infarction: a core dataset for monitoring standards of care. Royal College of Physicians of London, London

Birkhead JS, Walker L, Pearson M et al 2004 Improving care for patients with acute coronary syndromes: initial results from the National Audit of Myocardial Infarction Project (MINAP). Heart 90:1004–1009

Bjorklund E, Lindahl B, Stenestrand U 2004 Outcome of ST-elevation myocardial infarction treated with thrombolysis in the unselected population is vastly different from samples of eligible patients in a large-scale clinical trial. American Heart Journal 148:566–573

Department of Health 2000 National service framework for coronary heart disease. Department of Health, London

Dorsch MF, Lawrance RA, Sapsford RJ; EMMACE Study Group 2001 Poor prognosis of patients presenting with symptomatic myocardial infarction but without chest pain. Heart 86:494–498

Duncan P, Mackie F, Mackay F et al 2005 Use of statistical process control to support improvements in care for patients with acute myocardial infarction eligible for thrombolytic treatment: initial experience from two hospitals in England during 2002–03. Critical Pathways in Cardiology 4:21–25

French WJ 2000 Trends in acute myocardial infarction management: use of the National Registry of Myocardial Infarction in quality improvement. American Journal of Cardiology 85:5B–9B

Gamon R, Carolan K 2002 Reflections on the process of auditing myocardial infarction. European Journal of Cardiovascular Nursing 1:189–193

Hoekstra JW, Roe MT, Peterson ED et al 2005 Early glycoprotein IIb/IIIa inhibitor use for non-ST-segment elevation acute coronary syndrome: patient selection and associated treatment patterns. Academic Emergency Medicine 12:431–438

Mant J, Hicks N 1995 Detecting differences in the quality of care: the sensitivity of measures of process and outcome in treating acute myocardial infarction. British Medical Journal 311:793–796

National Assembly for Wales 2001 Tackling CHD in Wales: implementing through evidence. Welsh Assembly, Cardiff

Norris RM, Lowe D, Birkhead JS 2004 Can successful treatment of cardiac arrest be a performance indicator for hospitals? Resuscitation 60:263–269

Packham C, Gray D, Silcocks P 2000 Mortality of patients admitted with a suspected acute myocardial infarction in whom the diagnosis is not confirmed. European Heart Journal 21:206–212

Quinn T, Allan TF, Birkhead J, et al 2003 Impact of a region-wide approach to improving systems for heart attack care: the West Midlands Thrombolysis Project. European Journal of Cardiovascular Nursing 2:131–139

Scottish Executive 2002 Coronary heart disease and stroke strategy for Scotland. The Stationery Office, Edinburgh

Van de Werf F, Ardissino D, Betriu A et al 2003 The Task Force on the Management of Acute Myocardial Infarction of the European Society of Cardiology: management of acute myocardial infarction in patients presenting with ST-segment elevation. European Heart Journal 24:28–66

Van de Werf F, Gore JM, Avezum A et al 2005 Access to catheterisation facilities in patients admitted with acute coronary syndrome: multinational registry study. British Medical Journal 330:441

Weston CF 2004 Pre-hospital resuscitation: breathing life into a stale subject. Heart 90:1107–1109

Index

Notes: Entries in *italics* and **bold** represent figures and boxes/tables respectively. Abbreviations used as subentries and trial acronyms are as described in the front of the book.

A

Abciximab, properties/dosages, **140–141**
Actylise (alteplase), 102, **108–109**
acute coronary syndrome (ACS)
  burden of disease, 5
  care service models, 129
  complications, 65–74
    cardiac arrest, 66
    cardiogenic shock, 68–70
    heart failure, 66–68
    rhythmic disturbances *see*
      cardiac arrhythmias
    right ventricular infarction,
      53, 54, 70–71
    ventricular septal defect/
      rupture, 71
    see also specific complications
  definition, 4–5, *5*, *6*, 134
  ECG interpretation *see*
    electrocardiography
    (12-lead)
  measuring/improving quality of
    care, 153–160
  mortality, 5
  myocardial infarction *see*
    myocardial infarction (MI)
  pathophysiology, 4, *6*, 134
  unstable angina, 4, 5, 134, **136**

adenosine, **92–95**
  actions/uses, **92**
  cautions/contraindications, **93**
  dosage/route, **92, 94**
  side effects, **93, 95**
adjunctive therapy
  non-ST segment elevation, 137,
    140–141, 148–149
  percutaneous coronary
    interventions (PCI),
    129–130
  thrombolytic treatment, 111,
    112, 117, 118
  see also specific drugs
adrenaline (epinephrine), **86–87**
  actions/uses, **86**
  cautions/contraindications,
    87
  dosage/route, **86**
  in heart block, 83
  side effects, **87**
allergic reactions, thrombolytic
  treatment, 119–120
alteplase (Actylise), 102, **108–109**
ambulances, ECG, 9, 41
American College of Cardiology (ACC),
    PCI recommendations, 68
American Heart Association (AHA),
    PCI recommendations, 8, 68,
    128, 154

amiodarone, **88–92**
    actions/uses, **88, 90**
    cautions/contraindications, **89, 91**
    dosage/route, **88, 90, 92**
    side effects, **89, 91**
angina, unstable *see* unstable angina
angiograms, **125**
angioplasty, **125,** *126, 127*
anti-emetics, opiate analgesics and, 31
antifibrinolytic drugs, 118
antithrombotic drugs, **140–143**
    see also specific drugs
aprotinin, 118
arrhythmias *see* cardiac arrhythmias
aspirin
    as immediate priority, 28, 29–30
    NSTEMI, 137
    PCI and, 130
    properties/dosages, **140–141**
    thrombolysis and, 111
assessment *see* patient assessment
asystole, 96, *96, 97*
atenolol, properties/use of, **144–145**
atrial fibrillation, *77, 77*
atrioventricular (AV) block *see* heart
    block
atropine, **86–89**
    actions/uses, **86, 88**
    cautions/contraindications, **87,
    89**
    dosage/route, **86, 88**
    in heart block, 83
    side effects, **87, 89**
    in thrombolysis-induced
        hypotension, 119

B

balloon angioplasty, **125,** *126, 127*
beta-blockers
    contraindications, 148
    NSTEMI, 137, 148–149
    properties/use of, **144–145**

bisoprolol, properties/use of, **144–145**
bradycardia, 78, 80
    ECG, *81*
    management algorithm, *80*
    opiate analgesics and, 32
bundle branch block (BBB), 46, 58–59
    left, 58, 59
    mortality, 58, **58**
    right, 58

C

calcium channel blockers, NSTEMI,
    148
cardiac arrest, 66
    drugs used, **86–94**
        see also specific drugs
    ventricular arrhythmias and,
        84–85, 94–98, *96*
cardiac arrhythmias, 75–100
    adverse signs, 76
    bradycardia, 32, 78, 80, *80, 81*
    ECG monitoring, 76, *77, 78, 81,*
        82, 96, 97
    heart block *see* heart block
    management
        algorithms, *79, 80*
        drugs used, 83, **86–94**
            see also specific drugs
        heart block, 83–84
    narrow complex tachycardia, 77,
        77, 78, 79
    ventricular *see* ventricular
        arrhythmias
    see also specific arrhythmias
cardiac markers, **138–139**
    NSTEMI, 137
cardiogenic shock, 68–70
    predisposing conditions, 68, **69**
    prognosis, 69
    treatment, 70
carvedilol, properties/use of,
    144–145

Central Cardiac Audit Database, 155–156
chest electrodes, placement, 38–40, *40*
chest pain
 associated symptoms, 21–22
 character, 20–21
 duration/frequency, 21
 exacerbating/relieving factors, 21
 location, 19–20
 management, 29, 31–32
 non-ACS related, 21, **23**, 23–24
 radiation, 20
 rating scales, 20
 see also patient assessment
clinical audit, 155
 MINAP, 155–157
clopidogrel
 NSTEMI management, 137
 PCI and, 130
 properties/dosages, **140–141**
 STEMI management, 29–30, 111
communication, thrombolytic treatment, 103, 110
complete (third degree) heart block, 82–83, *83*
consciousness level, thrombolytic therapy, 117
'contact to thrombolysis' time, 10
coronary artery occlusion, 4, *127*
creatine kinase (CK), **138–139**

D

dalteparin, properties/dosages, **142–143**
DANAMI 2 trial, 129
defibrillation, timing and outcome, 6–7
diamorphine, 31
diltiazem, NSTEMI, 148
drug(s)
 antifibrinolytic, 118
 antithrombotic, **140–143**

arrhythmia management, 83, **86–94**
immediate priorities, 28, 29–30
STEMI management, 29–30
thrombolytic, 102–103, **104–109**, 116, 117
 adjunctive, 111, **112**, 118
see also specific drugs

E

ECG *see* electrocardiography (12-lead)
electrocardiography (12-lead), 35–44
 ACS manifestations, 46
 5 day mortality and, **47**
 arrhythmias *see* cardiac arrhythmias
 bundle branch block, 46, **58**, 58–59
 non-ST elevation *see* non-ST segment elevation MI (NSTEMI)
 ST elevation *see* ST segment elevation MI (STEMI)
 ambulance, 9, 41
 decision-making role, 36
 electrode placement, 38–40
 chest electrodes, 38–40, *40*
 limb electrodes, 38, *39*
 posterior leads, 40–42, *41*
 right-sided leads, 40–42, *41*
 immediate priority, 29, 30, 46
 interpretation, 36, 45–64
 orientation, 50–51, *51*
 ST segment, 47–50, *48, 49, 50*
 normal ECGs, *48, 49, 51*
 optimising quality, 37–38
 repeat, 36
 reperfusion criteria, **47**
 significant findings, 37
electrodes (ECG), placement, 38–40, *39, 40, 41*

emergency care, 3–16
    assessment *see* patient assessment
    immediate *see* immediate
        management
    measuring/improving quality,
        153–160
    pre-hospital, 9
    reperfusion *see* reperfusion
    systems delay, 9–10
    timing and outcome, 6–9, 18, 102
    *see also specific treatments/
        indications*
enoxaparin, properties/dosages,
    142–143
epinephrine *see* adrenaline
    (epinephrine)
eptifibatide, properties/dosages,
    142–143
ethnic differences, MI presentation,
    22
European Society of Cardiology (ESC),
    PCI recommendations, 8, 128,
    154

F

facilitated percutaneous coronary
    interventions (PCI), **126**
fibrinolytic therapy *see* thrombolytic
    treatment
first degree heart block, 81
'4 Ds' concept, 9–10

G

gender differences, MI presentation,
    20, 22
glycoprotein IIb/IIIa inhibitors
    NSTEMI, 137
    PCI and, 130
    properties/dosages, **140–143**
GRACE risk score, **136**

H

headaches, nitrates, 30
'heart attack' *see* myocardial infarction
    (MI)
heart block, 81–84
    first degree, 81, *82*
    second degree
        type 1 (Mobitz I; Wenkebach),
            81, *82*
        type 2 (Mobitz II), 82, *83*
    third degree (complete), 82–83, *83*
    treatment, 83–84
heart failure, 66–68
    classification, 67
    clinical features, 67
    management, 67–68
heparin
    cautions/contraindications, **112**
    NSTEMI, 137
    PCI and, 130
    side effects, **112**
    thrombolysis and, 111, 118
hypotension, thrombolytic treatment-
    induced, 119

I

idioventricular rhythm, 84, *85*
immediate management, 18, 27–34
    aspirin, 28, 29–30
    clopidogrel, 29–30
    ECG, 29, 30, 46
    IV access, 31
    nitrates, 28, 30
    oxygen, 28, 30
    pain relief, 29, 31–32
    priorities, 28–29
    vital signs, 28, 29
informed consent, thrombolysis, 103
interventional cardiology *see*
        percutaneous coronary
        interventions (PCI)

intracranial haemorrhage (ICH), 103, 118–119
    nifedipine 'bites' and, 118
    PCI *vs.* thrombolysis, 125
    risk factors, 103
intravenous access, as immediate priority, 31
ISIS II (1988) trial, 29, 111

J

'J point,' 48
junctional bradycardia, 80, *81*

K

Killip heart failure classification, 67

L

lactate dehydrogenase (LDH), **138–139**
left anterior descending (LAD) coronary artery occlusion, *127*
left bundle branch block (LBBB), 58, 59
left ventricular hypertrophy, 60
limb electrodes, placement, 38
low molecular weight heparin (LMWH), 111, 118
    properties/dosages, **142–143**

M

Metalyse *see* tenecteplase (TNK)
metoprolol, properties/use of, **144–145**
MINAP, 155–157
Mobitz I heart block (second degree type 1; Wenkebach), 81, *82*

Mobitz II heart block (second degree type 2), 82
morphine, 31
mortality, 5
    assessment, 155
    bundle branch block (BBB), 58, **58**
    ECG (12-lead) and 5 day mortality, **47**
    non-ST segment elevation MI (NSTEMI), 5, **58**, 134
    ST segment elevation MI (STEMI), 5, **58**
    thrombolytic treatment, 116
myocardial infarction (MI)
    cardiogenic shock after, **69**
    definition, 4, 5
    incidence, 5
    non-ST segment elevation *see* non-ST segment elevation MI (NSTEMI)
    pathophysiology, 4, *6*, 134
    presentation
        associated symptoms, 21–22
        atypical, 22–24, 28
        chest pain *see* chest pain
        ethnic differences, 22
        gender differences, 20, 22
    reperfusion *see* reperfusion
    ST segment elevation *see* ST segment elevation MI (STEMI)
    treatment
        adjuvant *see* adjunctive therapy
        defibrillation, 6–7
        drug therapy, 11, 29–30
        interventional *see* percutaneous coronary interventions (PCI)
        PCI *vs.* thrombolysis, 7, 11, 124–129
        thrombolysis *see* thrombolytic treatment
        timing, importance of, 7–10
        see also specific drugs/treatments

mortality (*Cont'd*)
myocardial ischaemia, 'silent,' 22
myocardial necrosis, 4
myoglobin, **138–139**

N

narrow complex tachycardia, 77, *77, 78, 79*
National Health Service (NHS) Data Directory, 156
National Heart Attack Alert program, '4 Ds model,' 9–10
National Service Framework (NSF), 7–8, **8,** 154
nifedipine, intracranial haemorrhage (ICH), 118
nitrates
 contraindications, 30
 immediate priority, 28, 30
 NSTEMI, 137, 148–149
 properties/use of, **144–147**
 side effects, 30
non-ST segment elevation MI (NSTEMI), 4, 11, 60–61, 133–152
 cardiac markers, 137, **138–139**
 ECG, 137
 high-risk patients, 134–135
  clinical characteristics, **135**
  identification/triage, 149
  risk scoring, 135, **136**
 incidence, 134
 low molecular weight heparin, 111
 management, 135–137
  adjunctive treatment, 137, 148–149
  antithrombotic, 137, **140–141**
  interventional, *148*
 mortality, 5, **58**

O

observational registries, 155–157
opiate analgesia, 31–32
outcome *vs.* process, 155
oxygen, immediate priority, 28, 30

P

pain relief, 29, 31–32
patient assessment, 17–26
 atypical presentations, 22–24, 28
 ECG *see* electrocardiography (12-lead)
 key questions, **19**
 non-verbal cues, 22
 prompts, **19,** 19–22
 speed/timing, 18
 see also chest pain
patient delays, 10
patient education, 10
percutaneous coronary interventions (PCI), 123–132
 adjunctive therapy, 129–130
 AHA/ESC recommendations, 8, 128, 154
 facilitated, **126**
 optimising patency, 129–130
 primary, 102, **126**
  cardiogenic shock, 69
  indications, 8–9
  outcomes, 124–129
  service models, 129
 'rescue,' 120, **126**
 standards, 154
 techniques, **125,** *126, 127, 128*
 thrombolysis *vs.,* 7, 11, 102, 124–129
  lower risk, 125
'preconditioning,' 21
pre-hospital emergency care, 9

primary percutaneous cardiac
interventions *see*
percutaneous coronary
interventions (PCI)
process *vs.* outcome data, 155
pulmonary rales, 67
pulseless electrical activity (PEA), 71,
97–98
pulseless ventricular tachycardia, 84,
94
P waves, asystole, 96, *96*, *97*

Q

QRS complex, 47

R

Rapilysin (reteplase), 102, **106–107**
reperfusion
dynamic nature, 117
ECG criteria, **47**
interventional cardiology
see percutaneous coronary
interventions (PCI)
thrombolysis *see* thrombolytic
treatment
timing and outcome, 7
'rescue' percutaneous coronary
interventions (PCI), 120,
126
respiratory depression, opiate
analgesics and, 31–32
reteplase (Rapilysin), 102,
106–107
right bundle branch block (RBBB),
58
right coronary artery occlusion (RCA),
51–53
right ventricular infarction (RVI),
70–71
cardiogenic shock after, **69**
inferior STEMI, 53, *54*, 70

S

second degree heart block
type 1 (Mobitz I; Wenkebach),
81, *82*
type 2 (Mobitz II), 82, *83*
'silent' myocardial ischaemia, 22
sinus bradycardia, 78, *81*
sinus tachycardia, 77
stents/stenting, **125**
drug-eluting, 129–130
insertion, *127*, *128*
Streptase *see* streptokinase
streptokinase, 102, **104–105**
allergic reactions, 119–120
hypotension and, 119
ST segment, 47–50
definition, 47–48
depression, 55, *56*, 56–57, *57*,
60, *61*
elevation
in MI *see* ST segment elevation
MI (STEMI)
non-MI, 59, **60**
measurement, 49, *50*
normal ECG, 48, *48*, *49*
in NSTEMI patients, 137
ST segment elevation MI (STEMI), 4
anterior MI, 53–55, *54*
anterolateral MI, 55
bradycardia, 78
clopidogrel, 29–30, 111
inferior MI, 51–53, *52*, *53*
acute, *53*, 56, *56*
right ventricular infarction,
53, *54*, 70
tall R waves, 56
interventional cardiology
see percutaneous coronary
interventions (PCI)
lateral (apical) MI, 55
measurement, 48–49, *49*, *50*,
51–57

ST segment elevation MI (STEMI) (*Cont'd*)
  mortality, 5, **58**
  posterior MI, 55–57, 56–57, 57
  thrombolysis *see* thrombolytic treatment
supraventricular arrhythmias, 77, 78
systems delay, 9–10

T

tachycardia
  management algorithm, 79
  narrow complex, 77, 77, 78
  ventricular, 84, 84, 85, 94–95
  see also specific arrhythmias
tenecteplase (TNK), 102, **104–107**
  dosage/administration, **105, 107**
third degree (complete) heart block, 82–83, 83
thrombolytic treatment, 101–114
  care during, 115–122
  communication, 103, 110
  complications, 103, 118–120
    allergic reactions, 119–120
    bleeding, 118–119
    hypotension, 119
    ICH *see* intracranial haemorrhage (ICH)
    recurrent ischaemia/ infarction/occlusion, 120
  'contact to thrombolysis' time, 10
  contraindications, **110**, 128
  drugs used, 102–103, **104–109**
    adjunctive, 111, **112**, 117, 118
    'third generation,' 116
    see also specific drugs
  initial management, 116–117
  mortality and outcome, 116
  observation during, 117–118
  PCI *vs.*, 7, 11, 102, 124–129
  pre-hospital, 9
  time dependency, 102

TIMI risk score, **136**
tirofiban, properties/dosages, **140–141**
tranexamic acid, 118
troponins, **138–139**
T wave, 47
  inversion, 60

U

unstable angina, 4, 5, 134
  risk assessment, **136**
  see also non-ST segment elevation MI (NSTEMI)

V

ventricular arrhythmias
  cardiac arrest associated, 84–85, 94–98
    non-shockable, 85, 96, 96–98, 97
    shockable, 84, 85, 94–95, 96
  not associated with cardiac arrest, 84, 85
  see also specific arrhythmias
ventricular fibrillation (VF), 84, 95, 96
ventricular septal defect/rupture, 71
ventricular tachycardia (VT), 84, 84, 85, 94–95
  characteristics, 85
  pulseless, 84, 94
  'salvos,' 94
verapamil, NSTEMI, 148
vital signs
  as immediate priority, 28, 29
  thrombolytic therapy, 117

W

Wenkebach heart block (Mobitz I; second degree type 1), 81, 82